THE BOOK OF NATURAL MEDICINE AND HERBAL REMEDIES

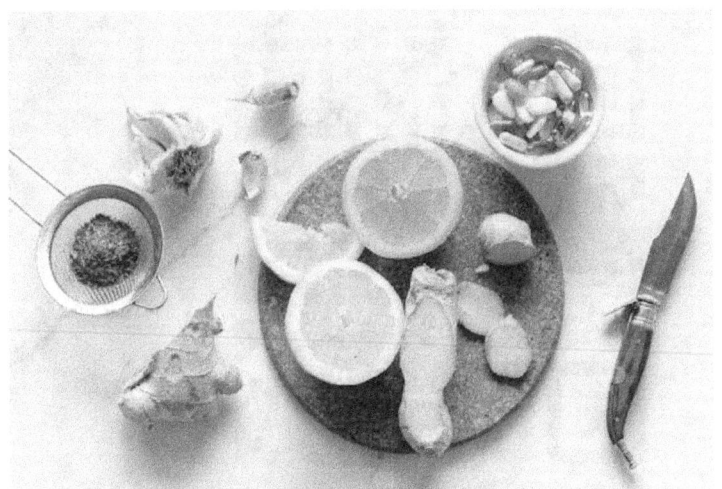

A Guide to Herbal Health and Cultivating Wellness

Raquel Williams

Copyright © 2024 by Raquel Williams

All rights reserved. This book or any portion thereof may not be reproduced or used in any manner whatsoever without the express written permission of the author except for the use of brief quotations in a book review.

My Author Central page

INTRODUCTION

In a world where synthetic drugs dominate, there lies an ancient wisdom waiting to be rediscovered—the healing magic of herbs and natural remedies. Welcome to "The Book of Natural Medicine and Herbal Remedies." Whether you're a seasoned herbalist or a curious seeker, this guide will take you on a transformative journey through the lush gardens of wellness.

Why Herbs Matter, imagine a world where vibrant health isn't just a distant dream but a daily reality. Herbs—those humble green guardians—hold the keys to vitality, resilience, and balance. From heart health to stress relief, they whisper secrets that modern medicine often overlooks. Beyond mere survival, we yearn for thriving. In these pages, we'll explore how to cultivate wellness from the roots up. Discover the art of blending herbs, creating tinctures, and brewing teas that dance with life force. Let's unlock the alchemy of well-being together.

From Garden to Heart, picture sun-kissed chamomile petals, the spicy warmth of ginger, and the soothing embrace of lavender. These aren't just ingredients; they're allies. Learn how to harness their power to nurture your heart, body, and soul. Our journey spans continents—from Ayurvedic wisdom in India to

Native American traditions, from Chinese herbalism to European folklore. Each culture contributes its unique tapestry of healing practices. Let's weave them into a holistic understanding of wellness.

Dive into chapters on heart-boosting herbs, stress resilience, and natural remedies for common ailments. Explore recipes, rituals, and time-tested practices. And remember, this isn't just a book; it's your invitation to a lifelong relationship with nature's medicine chest.

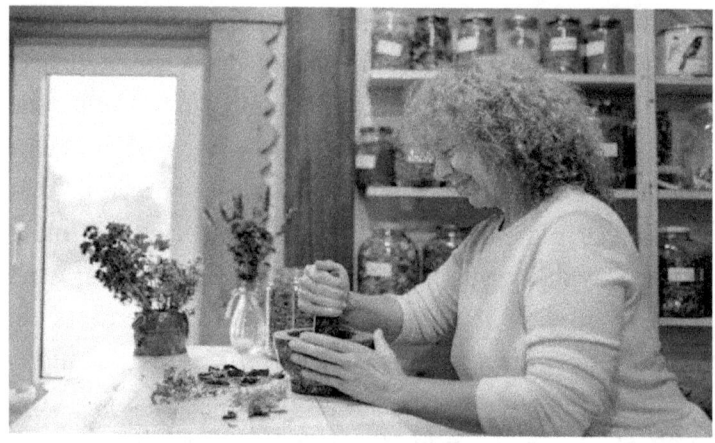

TABLE OF CONTENTS

INTRODUCTION   3
TABLE OF CONTENTS   5
  Overview of Natural Medicine and Herbal Remedies   **Error! Bookmark not defined.**
  Importance of Herbal Health   10
  History and Evolution of Herbal Medicine   13
  Inside the Book   20
  How to Use This Book   23
  Chapter 1: Foundations of Herbal Medicine   27
    Understanding Herbal Medicine   27
    Traditional vs. Modern Practices   35
    Safety and Precautions   40
  Chapter 2: Herbal Preparation Techniques   45
    Infusions and Teas   45
    Tinctures and Extracts   52
    Salves and Balms   66
    Essential Oils and Aromatherapy   72
  Chapter 3: Common Herbs and Their Uses   79
    Medicinal Properties of Herbs   79
    Culinary Herbs with Health Benefits   84
    Herbs for Immune Support   88
    Herbs for Digestive Health   93
  Chapter 4: Growing Your Own Herbs   99
    Choosing the Right Herbs for Your Garden   99
    Soil, Water, and Light Requirements   102
    Organic Gardening Practices   105
    Harvesting and Storing Herbs   109
  Chapter 5: Herbal Remedies for Common

Ailments   113
  Cold and Flu Relief   113
  Headache and Migraine Remedies   116
  Digestive Disorders and Solutions   120
  Skin Conditions and Treatments   123

Chapter 6: Herbal Remedies for Mental Health
  Herbs for Stress Relief   129
  Enhancing Mood with Herbs   131
  Herbal Solutions for Anxiety   132
  Herbal Support for Sleep Disorders   133

Chapter 7: Herbal Remedies for Women's Health   135
  Hormonal Balance   135
  Herbal Support for Menstruation and Menopause   136
  Fertility and Pregnancy   138
  Postpartum and Lactation Support   141

Chapter 8: Herbal Remedies for Men's Health
  Prostate Health   143
  Enhancing Libido and Stamina   144
  Herbs for Heart Health   146
  Managing Stress and Vitality   147

Chapter 9: Herbal Remedies for Children   149
  Safe Herbs for Children   149
  Remedies for Common Childhood Illnesses   151
  Herbal Support for Growth and Development
  Herbal Care for Skin and Allergies   155

Chapter 10: Herbal Detox and Cleansing   159
  Benefits of Detoxification   159
  Herbs for Liver Health   161

Herbal Support for Kidney and Urinary Health
Detoxifying Teas and Tonics 167
Chapter 11: Herbal Nutrition 170
- Nutrient-Rich Herbs 170
- Incorporating Herbs into Daily Diet 172
- Herbal Supplements and Powders 174
- Cooking with Herbs 176

Chapter 12: Herbal Remedies for Physical Fitness 178
- Pre-Workout Herbs 178
- Herbs for Muscle Recovery 180
- Enhancing Endurance with Herbs 183
- Herbal Solutions for Inflammation 186

Chapter 13: Herbal Remedies for Beauty and Skincare 190
- Natural Skincare Ingredients 190
- Herbal Hair Care 192
- Anti-Aging Herbal Remedies 194
- DIY Herbal Beauty Recipes 196

Chapter 14: Integrating Herbs into Daily Life 200
- Creating a Home Apothecary 200
- Herbal Remedies for Pets 206
- Sustainable Herbal Practices 207

Chapter 15: Advanced Herbal Medicine 212
- Clinical Applications of Herbal Medicine 212
- Herbal Formulations and Blends 214
- Research and Future of Herbal Medicine 216
- Resources and Further Reading 218

CONCLUSION 222

Overview of Natural Medicine and Herbal Remedies

"The Book of Natural Medicine and Herbal Remedies" explores ancient wisdom, revealing the healing power of plants. From echinacea to lavender, discover remedies that nurture well-being.

1. Echinacea: This flowering plant, also known as coneflower, has been used for centuries to treat various ailments. From Native American practices to modern times, echinacea has been associated with wound healing, sore throats, and upset stomachs. While research on its effectiveness is limited, some evidence suggests it may reduce the risk of catching a cold by up to 20%.

2. Ginseng: The roots of ginseng, particularly Asian (Panax ginseng) and American (Panax quinquefolius) varieties, have been steeped into teas or dried for powder. Although ancient wisdom praises ginseng for reducing inflammation, boosting immunity, and enhancing brain function, modern scientific evidence remains scarce. Still, its unique compounds, called ginsenosides, hold promise for neuroprotection, anticancer effects, and immune support.

3. **Oatmeal Face Mask:** For skin hydration, create an at-home face mask using oatmeal. Oatmeal acts as a humectant, helping your skin retain moisture. Mix hot water with oatmeal, Greek yoghourt, manuka honey, and egg white. Apply to your face for 10 minutes and rinse with lukewarm water.

4. **Exercise for Menopause:** As menopause symptoms hit, exercise becomes a powerful natural remedy. A mix of cardio and weight training keeps you feeling strong, boosts metabolism, and helps manage hormonal changes.

5. **Bleach as an Antibacterial:** Surprisingly, bleach serves as a natural antibacterial agent. It eliminates germs without contributing to antibiotic resistance. Use it wisely for cleaning and disinfection.

6. **Turmeric:** The golden spice, turmeric (Curcuma longa), contains curcumin—a potent anti-inflammatory compound. It's been used for centuries in Ayurvedic medicine to alleviate joint pain, support digestion, and boost immunity. Mix it into warm milk or add it to curries for a flavorful health boost.

7. **Lavender:** Beyond its delightful fragrance, lavender (Lavandula angustifolia) has calming properties. Use lavender essential oil for relaxation,

stress relief, and better sleep. A few drops on your pillow or in a warm bath can work wonders.

8. Peppermint: The invigorating scent of peppermint (Mentha × piperita) isn't just for candy. Peppermint tea soothes upset stomachs, eases headaches, and clears congestion. Plus, it's a natural breath freshener! Steep dried peppermint leaves for a refreshing cup.

9. Chamomile: When stress knocks at your door, chamomile (Matricaria chamomilla) tea invites calmness. It's a gentle sedative, perfect for winding down before bedtime. Sip on a cup of chamomile tea and let worries float away.

10. Aloe Vera: This succulent isn't just for sunburns. Aloe vera (Aloe barbadensis miller) gel is a skin superhero. It moisturises, soothes irritation, and promotes healing. Keep a potted aloe plant handy for emergencies.

Importance of Herbal Health

Herbal health is a timeless approach to wellness that harnesses the natural potency of plants to promote physical and mental well-being. By utilising herbal remedies, individuals can tap into centuries-old knowledge to support their body's natural healing processes. Here's a compelling explanation for the importance of herbal health.

1. **Embracing Nature's Pharmacy:** Herbs have been nature's pharmacy for thousands of years, offering a bounty of remedies that support health and wellness. They are the foundation of many modern medicines and continue to be a valuable resource for those seeking natural treatment options.

2. **Synergy of Compounds:** Unlike synthetic drugs that often isolate specific compounds, herbs contain a symphony of chemical constituents that work together synergistically. This complexity allows them to address multiple facets of a health issue, often improving efficacy and reducing the risk of side effects.

3. **Adaptogenic Properties:** Many herbs are adaptogens, which means they help the body adapt to stress and exert a normalising effect upon bodily processes. This is important in our fast-paced world, where chronic stress can lead to a host of health problems.

4. **Cultural and Historical Significance:** Herbal medicine is steeped in history and tradition, with each culture having its own herbal practices. By learning about and using herbal remedies, we honour

the wisdom of our ancestors and preserve important cultural heritage.

5. Personal Empowerment: Learning about and using herbs can empower individuals to take an active role in their health. It fosters a sense of autonomy and connection with one's health journey, encouraging proactive and informed health choices.

6. Environmental Stewardship: Cultivating and using herbs can promote environmental health. Many herbs can be grown sustainably and have a lower environmental footprint compared to mass-produced pharmaceuticals.

7. Economic Viability: The herbal health market is growing as people seek out natural alternatives to conventional medicine. This presents an opportunity for entrepreneurs and farmers to tap into a market that values sustainability, health, and wellness. By delving into the world of herbal health, your book will not only serve as a guide to personal wellness but also as a beacon for sustainable living and a testament to the enduring power of natural medicine.

8. Skin and Hair Care: Herbs like aloe vera, lavender, and rosemary offer natural solutions for skin and hair care, often found in beauty products for their healing and restorative properties.

9. Heart Health: Herbs like hawthorn and garlic have been shown to support heart health by improving circulation and reducing blood pressure. Antioxidant-rich herbs can combat free radicals, reducing the signs of aging and promoting longevity.

10. Culinary Uses: Beyond health benefits, herbs enhance the flavour of food, encouraging a healthy and enjoyable eating experience. The practice of growing, harvesting, and using herbs can foster a sense of community and connection to nature.

History and Evolution of Herbal Medicine

The history and evolution of herbal medicine is a rich and diverse tapestry that spans across various cultures and millennia. Here's a brief overview.

Ancient Beginnings: Herbal medicine has its roots in the ancient world, with evidence of its use in Sumerian and Egyptian civilizations. The Ebers Papyrus, dating back to 1550 BCE, is one of the oldest surviving medical texts and includes many herbal remedies. Traditional Chinese Medicine (TCM). In China, the use of herbs is well-documented in the classic text "The Divine Farmer's Herb-Root Classic" (Shennong Bencao Jing), written around 200-250 CE. TCM has developed a sophisticated approach to diagnosing and treating illnesses with herbs over thousands of years.

Ayurveda: Originating in India, Ayurveda is another ancient system of medicine that utilises herbs. Texts like the Charaka Samhita and the Sushruta Samhita describe the medicinal properties of various plants and are foundational to Ayurvedic practice.

Greek and Roman Influence: The works of Hippocrates and Galen are significant in the Western tradition of herbal medicine. They both emphasised the importance of balance and the use of natural remedies, including herbs.

Middle Ages and Renaissance: During this period, monasteries became centers for the study of herbal medicine. The "Materia Medica" by Dioscorides was a key text that influenced herbal knowledge in Europe for over 1,500 years.

Modern Era: The 19th and 20th centuries saw a shift towards synthetic pharmaceuticals, but there has been a resurgence of interest in herbal medicine as people seek more natural and holistic approaches to health.

Current Trends: Today, herbal medicine is a blend of traditional knowledge and modern scientific research. It's recognized as a form of complementary and alternative medicine, with ongoing studies into the efficacy and mechanisms of herbal remedies.Ancient

Civilizations:
1. **Mesopotamia:** The Sumerians compiled lists of plants on clay tablets, some of which were used for medicinal purposes. These early pharmacopoeias laid the groundwork for future herbal compendiums.

2. **Egypt:** The Ebers Papyrus not only lists remedies but also spells and incantations to ward off spirits believed to cause diseases. It reflects the intertwined nature of magic and medicine in ancient practices.

3. **Traditional Chinese Medicine:** Herbal Classics, TCM is known for its "Three Treasures" concept (Qi, Jing, Shen) and the use of herbs to balance these energies. The Shennong Bencao Jing categorises hundreds of medicinal substances and their effects on the body's harmony.

4. **Herbalists:** Figures like Paracelsus challenged Galenic medicine and emphasised the use of chemicals found in nature, which included plants, for healing. 18th and 19th Centuries: Scientific

Revolution: The study of botany became more scientific, leading to the isolation of compounds like morphine from plants, which paved the way for modern pharmacology. 20th Century to Present.

1. **Regulation and Research:** With the rise of synthetic drugs, herbal medicine faced scrutiny and regulation. However, research into plant-based compounds has continued, with many modern drugs being derived from plants.

2. **Global Integration:** The World Health Organization recognizes traditional medicine and supports integrating it into national health systems, reflecting a global appreciation for herbal remedies.

3. **Contemporary Practice:** Evidence-Based Herbalism, There's a growing emphasis on clinical trials and scientific evidence to support the efficacy and safety of herbal treatments.

The Dawn of Herbal Medicine: Roots in Antiquity In the cradle of civilization, the fertile crescent of Mesopotamia, the earliest humans discovered the healing properties of plants. This nascent understanding laid the foundation for a practice that would span across cultures and epochs. The Sumerians, with their cuneiform tablets, documented the use of thyme, licorice, and mustard plants, among others, for ailments ranging from coughs to wounds. Moving to the banks of the Nile, the ancient Egyptians furthered this herbal knowledge. The Ebers Papyrus, a treasure trove of medical wisdom, lists over 850 natural remedies, including garlic for heart conditions and aloe vera for skin health. These remedies were often accompanied by prayers and incantations, reflecting a world where the spiritual and physical were deeply intertwined.

The Philosophers and Physicians: Greco-Roman Contributions The Greeks, led by the likes of Hippocrates, the father of medicine, began to systematise the knowledge of herbs. Hippocrates' humoral theory suggested that health was a state of balance among the body's fluids, and herbs were one way to restore equilibrium. His contemporary, Theophrastus, is often dubbed the father of botany for his extensive work in plant classification. In Rome, Galen built upon Hippocratic medicine, and his texts would dominate Western medical thought for centuries. His methodical approach to using herbs based on their cooling or warming properties influenced the development of pharmacopoeias across the Roman Empire.

The Silk Road to Enlightenment: Asian Traditions As the Silk Road bridged East and West, so too did it facilitate the exchange of medicinal plant knowledge. In China, the legendary Shennong, the Divine Farmer, was said to have tasted hundreds of herbs, imparting his knowledge in the "Shennong Bencao Jing." This text categorised herbs into three classes based on their properties and toxicity, a classification system still influential in Traditional Chinese Medicine (TCM) today. In the Indian subcontinent, Ayurveda, the "science of life," emerged as a holistic system where herbs played a crucial role. Texts like the "Charaka Samhita" and "Sushruta Samhita" detailed the properties of plants like turmeric and ashwagandha, which are still used today to balance the doshas—vata, pitta, and kapha—and maintain health.

The Medieval Garden: Monasteries as Centers of Healing With the fall of the Roman Empire, much of the classical knowledge of herbs might have been lost if not for the monasteries of Europe. Monks and nuns became the keepers of herbal wisdom, cultivating gardens where they grew plants like sage, chamomile, and lavender. Hildegard of Bingen, a Benedictine abbess, wrote extensively on the medicinal uses of plants, combining her spiritual insights with practical herbal knowledge. Herbalists like Nicholas Culpeper democratised herbal knowledge, making it accessible to the common folk and challenging the medical establishment.

The Age of Reason: Science and Synthesis The Enlightenment and the subsequent scientific revolution brought a more empirical approach to understanding herbs. Botanists like Carl Linnaeus developed classification systems that are still in use today. The isolation of morphine from opium poppies in the early 19th century marked the beginning of modern pharmacology, where the active principles of herbs began to be extracted and synthesised.

The Modern Era: A Return to Roots Despite the rise of synthetic pharmaceuticals, the 20th century saw a resurgence in the interest in herbal medicine. The counterculture movement of the 1960s and 1970s, with its emphasis on natural living, and the holistic health movement, brought herbal medicine back into the public consciousness. Today, herbal medicine is a global phenomenon, blending traditional wisdom with scientific research. The World Health Organization supports the integration of traditional herbal practices into modern medical systems, recognizing their value and potential for wellness.

Inside the Book

This structure offers readers a clear and informative path through the world of herbal medicine, from the foundational knowledge to practical applications. It's designed to be both educational and engaging, providing valuable insights for both beginners and seasoned herbal enthusiasts. Inside This Book, You Will Discover,

1. Foundations of Herbal Medicine: Dive into the ancient wisdom and modern science that form the bedrock of herbal medicine. Uncover the healing power of plants and learn how to harness this knowledge responsibly and effectively. This section will guide you through the history, principles, and evidence-based practices that ensure the safe use of herbal remedies.

2. Herbal Preparation Techniques: Gain proficiency in creating a variety of herbal preparations with step-by-step instructions. From soothing teas and potent tinctures to healing salves and aromatic essential oils, you'll learn the methods to extract the full spectrum of therapeutic benefits from each herb. This hands-on guide will empower you to transform raw plant materials into remedies that can support health and well-being.

3. Common Herbs and Their Uses: Embark on a journey through the herbal kingdom with a detailed exploration of the most widely used herbs. Discover the unique properties of each plant, including their indications, modes of action, and synergistic effects. This comprehensive directory will provide insights into herbs for bolstering the immune system, promoting digestive harmony, enhancing mental clarity, and much more.

4. Growing Your Own Herbs: Experience the satisfaction of planting and nurturing your own herbal garden. Whether you have a sprawling backyard or a small balcony space, this section will guide you through selecting the right herbs for your environment, implementing sustainable gardening techniques, and ensuring a bountiful harvest. Learn the secrets to preserving the vitality of your herbs through proper harvesting, drying, and storage methods.

4. Herbal Therapies for Mental and Emotional Well-being: Explore the world of adaptogens, nervines, and other herbs that support mental health. Learn how herbal remedies can be used to alleviate stress, anxiety, and improve sleep, complementing traditional therapies.

21

5, Herbal First Aid: Discover how to create an herbal first aid kit equipped with natural remedies for cuts, bruises, burns, and common ailments. This section will provide practical advice on how to use herbs in emergency situations and for everyday health concerns.

6. The Art of Herbal Formulation: Delve into the art and science of combining herbs to enhance their healing properties. Understand the principles of synergy and how to formulate effective herbal blends for a variety of health conditions.

7. Cultural Traditions in Herbal Medicine: Take a global tour of herbal practices across different cultures. From the Ayurvedic herbs of India to the traditional remedies of Native American tribes, this section celebrates the diversity and wisdom of global herbal traditions.

8. Modern Research and Future Directions: Stay informed about the latest scientific research on herbal medicine, including clinical trials and studies on phytochemicals. Look ahead to the future of herbalism and the potential for new discoveries and applications.

How to Use This Book

Welcome to a journey of herbal discovery and natural wellness. "The Book of Natural Medicine and Herbal Remedies" is designed to be both a comprehensive guide and a practical companion on your path to understanding and using herbal medicine.

1. Start with the Basics: Begin by reading the Foundations of Herbal Medicine to build a solid understanding of the principles that underpin herbal practice. This knowledge will support your learning as you delve deeper into the book.

2. Follow the Instructions: As you explore the Herbal Preparation Techniques use the detailed instructions as a step-by-step guide to creating your own remedies. The clear, concise directions are there to ensure your success and safety.

3. Refer to the Herb Directory: The Common Herbs and Their Uses, section is a resource you can come back to time and again. Use it to look up specific herbs, learn about their benefits, and find out how to incorporate them into your health regimen.

4. Get Your Hands Dirty: When you're ready to start your own herb garden, the Growing Your Own

Herbs, chapter will be your go-to guide. It's filled with practical tips for gardeners of all levels, from novice to expert.

5. Expand Your Knowledge: The additional sections on mental well-being, first aid, and cultural traditions offer deeper dives into specialised areas of herbal medicine. Use these chapters to broaden your understanding and appreciation of the herbal world.

6. Keep it Within Reach: Keep this book in a place where you can easily access it, whether that's on your kitchen shelf for quick reference while cooking or on your bedside table for evening reading.

7. Take Notes: Don't be afraid to make this book your own. Use the margins to jot down notes, highlight passages that resonate with you, and bookmark pages you want to revisit.

8. Practise Mindfully: As you put the teachings of this book into practice, do so with mindfulness and respect for the power of plants. Remember that herbal medicine is about balance and harmony with nature.

9. Share the Knowledge: Herbal medicine is a communal practice. Share what you've learned with friends and family, and encourage them to join you on this path to herbal health.

10. Stay Curious: Use the "Modern Research and Future Directions" section to stay informed about the latest developments in herbal medicine. Let your curiosity lead you to new studies, workshops, and seminars.

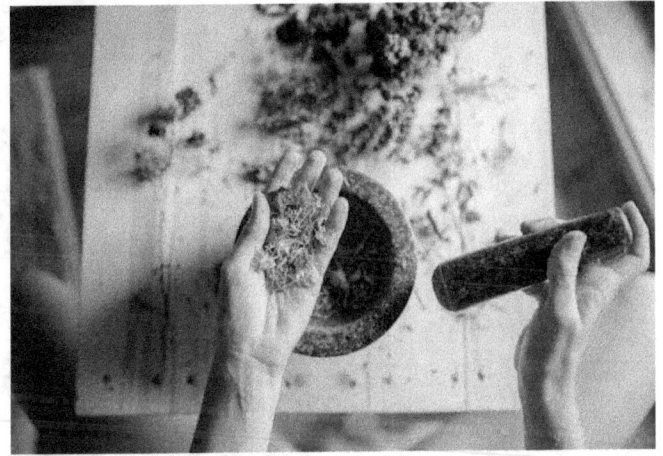

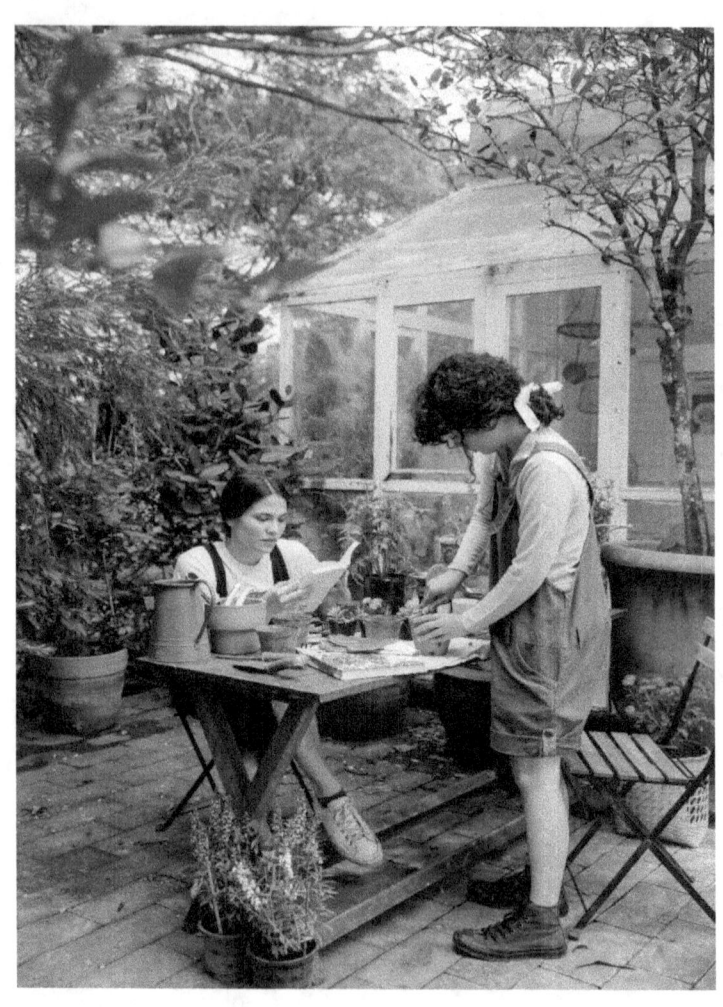

Chapter 1: Foundations of Herbal Medicine

Understanding Herbal Medicine

Herbal medicine, also known as phytotherapy or botanical medicine, involves using a plant's seeds, berries, roots, leaves, bark, or flowers for medicinal purposes. The practice is deeply rooted in the belief that natural substances, particularly plants, have the power to heal and balance the body. Here's a detailed explanation of the key concepts and practices in herbal medicine.

The Philosophy of Herbal Medicine: Herbal medicine is founded on the principle that plants contain natural substances that can promote health and alleviate illness. The holistic approach of herbal medicine looks at the individual as a whole, considering their physical, emotional, and spiritual well-being.

Active Constituents: Plants produce a variety of biochemical compounds that serve different functions, such as protection from insects or fungi. These compounds, when used in humans, can have therapeutic effects. For example, the salicylic acid found in willow bark is the basis for aspirin.

Synergy in Herbal Blends: Unlike conventional medicine, which often isolates individual compounds, herbal medicine frequently uses whole plants or blends to take advantage of the synergy between various plant constituents. This synergy may enhance the therapeutic effects and reduce the risk of side effects.

Herbal Preparations: Herbs can be prepared in several ways, including

1. Teas or Infusions: These are the most common and well-known herbal preparations. To make them, you steep leaves or flowers from herbs in hot water. This allows the active compounds and flavours to dissolve into the water, resulting in a soothing and flavorful beverage. You can drink herbal teas for their potential health benefits or simply for enjoyment.

2. Decoctions: Decoctions are similar to infusions, but they are used to extract active compounds from tougher plant materials like roots, bark, or berries. Instead of steeping in hot water, you simmer or boil these materials to break them down and release their compounds into the water. Decoctions often have a more concentrated taste and are consumed for their therapeutic effects.

3. Tinctures: Tinctures are liquid extracts made by soaking herbs in alcohol or glycerin. This process draws out and preserves the active ingredients from the herbs. Tinctures are typically more concentrated than teas or decoctions, so you only need a small amount to experience the therapeutic effects. They can be taken directly by mouth or added to water or other beverages.

4. Salves and Ointments: These herbal preparations are used topically to soothe, protect, or heal the skin. Salves and ointments are made by combining herbal extracts with a base of waxes, fats, or oils. This creates a semi-solid mixture that can be easily applied to the skin. Herbal salves and ointments can be used for a variety of skin issues, such as minor cuts, scrapes, rashes, and irritation.

Dosage and Administration: The effectiveness of herbal medicine depends on the correct dosage and administration. Factors such as the part of the plant used, the time of harvest, and the method of preparation all play a role in the potency of the remedy.

Safety and Efficacy: While many herbs are safe when used appropriately, some can cause side effects or interact with other medications. It's important to understand the safety profile of each herb and to consult with a healthcare professional, especially for serious conditions.

Evidence-Based Herbalism: Modern herbal practitioners combine traditional knowledge with scientific research. Clinical studies on herbs help to validate their use and understand the mechanisms behind their effects.

Cultural and Traditional Contexts: Herbal medicine is practised differently across cultures, with each tradition having its own set of herbs and methods. For example, Traditional Chinese Medicine and Ayurveda have unique diagnostic systems and herbal formulations.

Sustainability and Ethical Sourcing: With the growing demand for herbal products, sustainable cultivation and ethical sourcing have become crucial to protect plant species from overharvesting and to ensure the quality of herbal remedies.

Integrative Approach: Many practitioners of herbal medicine advocate for an integrative approach, where herbal therapies complement conventional medical treatments. This collaboration aims to provide a more comprehensive care model for patients.

The Science Behind Herbs

In the realm of natural health, the allure of herbal medicine is not just in its tradition but also in its scientific substantiation. The science behind herbs is a fascinating confluence of botany, chemistry, and medicine that reveals how plants can be potent allies in our quest for wellness. Here's a detailed explanation that not only underscores the credibility of herbal medicine but also highlights its marketable potential.

Phytochemistry: The Chemical Language of Plants
Plants synthesise an array of chemical compounds known as phytochemicals, which they use to protect themselves from predators and diseases, and to attract pollinators. When these phytochemicals interact with the human body, they can promote healing and support health. For instance, the curcumin in turmeric is a powerful anti-inflammatory agent, while the ginsenosides in ginseng boost energy and resilience.

Pharmacognosy: From Plant to Prescription
Pharmacognosy is the study of medicinal drugs derived from plants and other natural sources. This discipline involves identifying, extracting, and analysing bioactive compounds that can be developed into medications. Many of today's pharmaceuticals have their origins in plant compounds, such as the heart medication digoxin from foxglove and the cancer drug paclitaxel from the Pacific yew tree.

Clinical Trials: Validating Efficacy The true test of any medicinal herb lies in clinical trials that evaluate its efficacy and safety. Rigorous studies help to confirm the therapeutic benefits claimed by traditional use. For example, St. John's Wort has been extensively studied and is now widely accepted as an effective treatment for mild to moderate depression.

Herbal Synergy: The Entourage Effect Unlike synthetic drugs that typically contain a single active ingredient, herbal remedies often include a complex mix of phytochemicals that work together to enhance their therapeutic effects—a phenomenon known as the entourage effect. This holistic approach can offer a broader spectrum of action and reduce the likelihood of resistance or side effects.

Standardisation: Ensuring Consistency To make herbal medicine a reliable and profitable venture, standardisation is key. It ensures that herbal products contain a consistent level of active ingredients, making them dependable for consumers and attractive for retailers. Standardised extracts are the gold standard in the herbal supplement industry.

Regulation and Quality Control: Building Trust Regulatory frameworks, such as those enforced by the FDA in the United States or the EMA in Europe, help to build consumer trust by ensuring that herbal products are safe, of high quality, and labelled accurately. This oversight is crucial for maintaining the integrity of the market and protecting public health.

Market Trends: Riding the Wave of Wellness The global herbal supplement market is booming, driven by an increasing consumer focus on wellness and natural products. Capitalising on this trend requires not only a solid understanding of the science behind herbs but also savvy marketing that communicates the benefits and research-backed credentials of herbal remedies.

Educating Consumers: Knowledge as Power An informed customer is a loyal customer. Providing clear, science-based information about the efficacy and safety of herbal products empowers consumers to make educated choices, fostering a sustainable and profitable relationship between producers and consumers.

The Future of Herbal Science: Innovation and Discovery The field of herbal medicine is ripe with potential for new discoveries. Ongoing research into lesser-known plants and novel compounds promises to expand the horizons of natural health products, offering exciting opportunities for growth in the industry.

Adaptogenic Herbs: Nature's Stress Relievers have gained prominence for their ability to enhance the body's resistance to stressors. Here's how they work.
1. **Homeostasis:** Adaptogens support the body's ability to achieve homeostasis, the state of equilibrium between different physiological processes.
2. **HPA Axis Regulation:** They modulate the hypothalamic-pituitary-adrenal (HPA) axis, which governs our stress response. Stress Protection: By regulating cortisol levels, adaptogens can help the body cope with stress, fatigue, and anxiety.
Examples: Some well-known adaptogens include Ashwagandha, Rhodiola Rosea, and Ginseng.

Antioxidant Herbs: Combating Oxidative Stress Antioxidants are compounds that inhibit oxidation, a chemical reaction that can produce free radicals, leading to cell damage. Antioxidant herbs are rich in these compounds and offer protection against
1. **oxidative stress:** Free Radical Scavengers: Antioxidant herbs contain compounds like flavonoids and polyphenols that neutralise free radicals. Chronic

2. Disease Prevention: By reducing oxidative stress, these herbs may help prevent chronic diseases such as heart disease and cancer.

Examples: Herbs like Turmeric, Green Tea, and Holy Basil are potent sources of antioxidants.

Traditional vs. Modern Practices

Herbal medicine is an art form that has evolved over thousands of years, yet it remains grounded in the wisdom of the past. In today's health and wellness market, the juxtaposition of traditional and modern practices of herbal medicine offers a unique point.

Traditional Herbal Medicine:
Rooted in Culture: Traditional herbal medicine practices are deeply ingrained in various cultures and societies, with knowledge passed down through generations. These practices are characterised by a holistic approach to healing, emphasising the balance between mind, body, and spirit.

Local Flora: Traditional herbal medicine practices often rely on locally available plants, which not only promotes self-sufficiency and local economy but also helps preserve traditional knowledge about indigenous flora.

Spiritual Elements: Many traditional systems incorporate spiritual or energetic aspects that address an individual's overall well-being. This holistic approach can be appealing to those seeking a more comprehensive approach to healthcare.

Customised Treatments: Traditional herbal medicine practitioners often tailor remedies to an individual's specific needs and conditions, taking into account their physical, emotional, and environmental factors. This personalised approach can create a more effective and satisfactory experience for consumers.

Modern Herbal Medicine:
Scientific Validation: Modern herbal medicine practices increasingly rely on evidence-based research to validate the efficacy and safety of herbal remedies. This scientific validation appeals to consumers who value empirical data and proof of effectiveness.

Standardisation: Standardising extracts ensures consistent active ingredient levels, making it easier for consumers to choose products that meet their specific needs. Standardisation also enables more accurate dosing and safety assessments, enhancing consumer trust.

Globalisation: The global marketplace offers access to a wide variety of plants and compounds, allowing for the development of innovative and diverse herbal products. This diversity can cater to a broader range of consumer preferences and needs.

Integration with Conventional Medicine: Integrating herbal treatments with conventional medical practices allows for a more comprehensive approach to healthcare. Consumers seeking complementary and alternative therapies will appreciate the benefits of an integrative approach.

Consumer Appeal: By combining traditional wisdom and modern science, herbal medicine can provide consumers with a powerful and appealing combination of authenticity and efficacy.

Educational Marketing: Sharing the historical context of herbal remedies alongside current research findings helps consumers understand the depth and value of herbal medicine, leading to more informed and engaged customers.

Quality Assurance: Highlighting the rigorous quality control measures used in modern herbal medicine practices reassures consumers of product safety and effectiveness, fostering loyalty and trust.

Personalization: Offering personalised herbal consultations or formulations creates a unique and customised wellness experience, appealing to consumers seeking tailored solutions.

Wellness Lifestyle: Positioning herbal medicine as part of a broader wellness lifestyle attracts consumers who value natural and holistic approaches to health.

Subscription Services: Implementing a subscription model provides customers with a convenient way to maintain their wellness routine, ensuring consistent engagement and revenue.

Workshops and Education: Educational opportunities, such as workshops or online courses, foster a dedicated customer base eager to invest in their health and deepen their understanding of herbal medicine.

The Educational Journey:
Storytelling: Utilise the rich history of herbal medicine as a storytelling tool to engage customers. Captivate your audience with narratives about ancient healers, traditional ceremonies, and the rediscovery of old remedies in modern science.

Transparency: Be transparent about sourcing, preparation methods, and the scientific backing of herbal products. This builds trust and positions your brand as a reputable source in the market.

Product Diversification: Cater to both traditionalists and modern health enthusiasts by offering a range of products. For example, sell whole herbs for those who prefer traditional preparations, and standardised capsules for customers who prioritise convenience and consistency.

Collaborations: Partner with practitioners of traditional herbal medicine, such as Ayurvedic doctors or Traditional Chinese Medicine practitioners, to create authentic products and experiences.

Sustainability: Emphasise sustainable practices in sourcing and production to attract eco-conscious consumers who are willing to pay a premium for environmentally friendly and ethically sourced products.

Expanding the Market:
Demographic Targeting: Tailor marketing campaigns to different demographics. Older generations may resonate more with traditional aspects, while younger consumers might be attracted to the modern, scientific approach.

Global Reach: Utilise e-commerce to reach a global audience. Offer detailed information and virtual consultations to provide a personalised experience to customers worldwide.

Community Building: Create a community around herbal medicine by hosting forums, social media groups, or membership clubs. This fosters loyalty and word-of-mouth marketing.

Innovation in Herbal Medicine:
Research Partnerships: Engage in partnerships with academic institutions to conduct research on herbal remedies. This adds credibility to your products and contributes to the scientific community.
Technology Integration: Use technology to enhance the customer experience, such as apps that track wellness progress or offer personalised herbal recommendations based on AI algorithms.

Safety and Precautions

When delving into the world of herbal medicine, safety is paramount. While herbs are natural, they are not inherently without risk. Here's a detailed guide on safety and precautions to consider.

Understanding Herb-Drug Interactions: Herb-drug interactions occur when herbs and medications are used together, potentially leading to undesirable effects. This can happen because certain herbs and drugs may have similar or opposing actions in the body. These interactions can affect drug absorption, metabolism, or excretion, which can either increase or decrease the drug's efficacy or the herb's potency. It is crucial to consult a healthcare professional before combining herbal remedies with other medications.

Recognizing Quality and Purity: To ensure the quality and purity of herbal products, look for certifications from reputable organisations. These certifications typically involve rigorous testing to confirm the identity, potency, and purity of the herbal product. It is also essential to be aware of the potential for contamination with pesticides, heavy metals, or adulterants, which can pose serious health risks.

Dosage and Administration: Adhering to recommended dosages is vital, as taking too much of an herb can be harmful, even if it is generally considered safe. It is also essential to understand the proper way to administer herbs, as some are meant to be consumed orally, while others should only be used topically.

Side Effects and Allergies: Be aware of potential side effects of herbs, which can range from mild to severe, depending on the herb and the individual. Allergic reactions to herbs are also possible, so caution should be taken, especially when trying a new herb.

Special Populations: Some herbs may not be safe for certain individuals, such as pregnant or breastfeeding women, as they may pose risks to the baby. Children and the elderly may also be more sensitive to the effects of herbs, so it may be necessary to adjust dosages accordingly.

Sustainability and Ethical Harvesting: Overharvesting can lead to environmental damage and the loss of biodiversity, making it essential to support sustainable harvesting practices. Ethical sourcing ensures that herbs are harvested responsibly and without causing harm to the environment or local communities.

Staying Informed: Stay updated on the latest research concerning herbal safety and efficacy, as new information may become available over time. Additionally, report any adverse reactions to healthcare providers or regulatory bodies to help ensure the safety of herbal products for all consumers.

Legal and Regulatory Considerations: Understand the legal status of herbs in your region, as regulations may differ depending on whether an herb is classified as a dietary supplement or a drug. Proper labelling, including ingredients, dosages, and warnings, is also vital for ensuring that consumers have the information they need to make informed decisions about using herbal products.

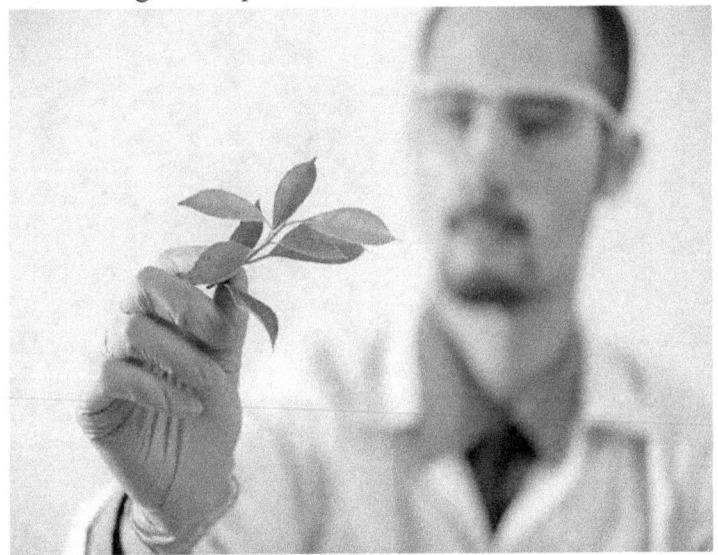

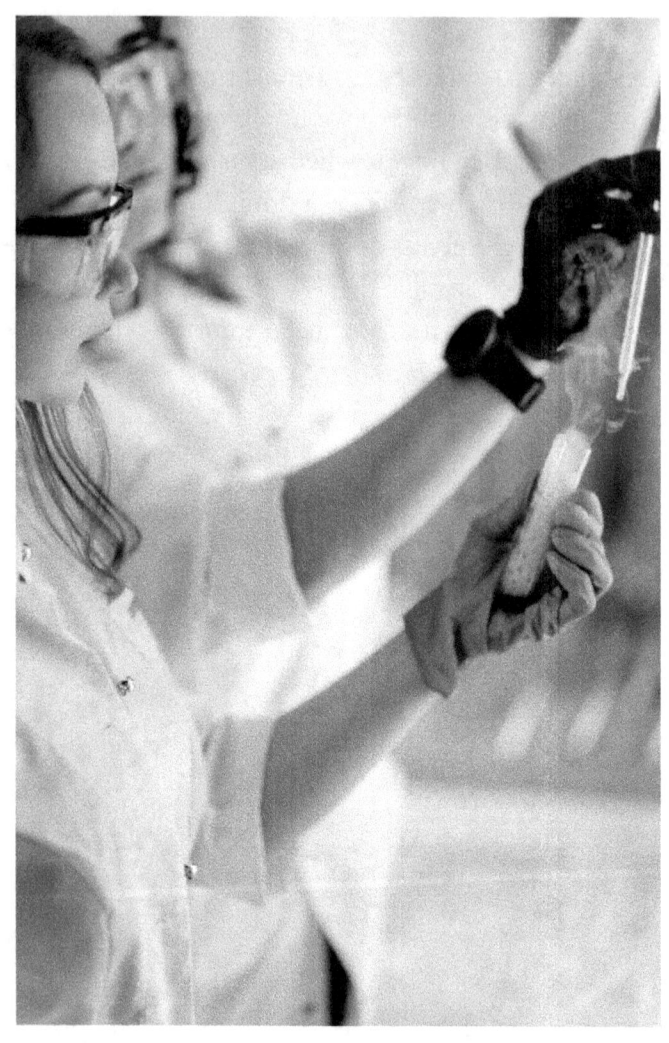

Chapter 2: Herbal Preparation Techniques

Infusions and Teas

Infusions and teas are among the most ancient and widely practiced methods of extracting the healing properties of herbs. They are cherished not only for their medicinal benefits but also for the ritual and comfort they provide. This is typically done with delicate parts of the plant—leaves, flowers, or aromatic stems—due to their volatile compounds and essential oils that can be lost under intense heat or prolonged boiling. Here's a detailed exploration of these herbal brews.

The Process:
Steeping: To make an infusion, the plant material is steeped in hot water for a specific period, usually between 5 to 15 minutes. The water should be just off the boil, around 90°C to 95°C (194°F to 203°F), to avoid destroying the herb's delicate constituents.Infusions and teas are two popular methods of preparing and consuming herbs, each offering a unique way to extract the beneficial compounds from plants.

Ratio: The standard ratio for making an infusion is about one teaspoon of dried herb or one tablespoon of fresh herb per cup of water. This ensures the right balance of strength and flavour, tailored to the herb's potency and intended use.

Covering: During steeping, it's essential to cover the vessel to prevent the escape of volatile oils and aromatic compounds. This not only preserves the therapeutic benefits of the herbs but also enhances the infusion's flavour and aroma.
Example: Use a lid, a plate, or even a dedicated tea cover to seal the vessel while the herbs steep.

Benefits of Infusions
1. Gentle Extraction: Infusions gently coax out the phytochemicals from herbs, preserving their active ingredients' integrity. This method avoids the harsh processes that can degrade sensitive compounds, ensuring that you receive the full therapeutic benefits.
Example: An infusion of chamomile flowers retains its soothing properties, helping to relax and promote sleep.

Hydration: Infusions provide a hydrating way to consume herbs, contributing to overall health. They offer an excellent alternative to plain water, adding

both flavour and health benefits to your hydration routine.
Example: Drinking a lavender infusion can be both refreshing and calming, supporting mental well-being while hydrating.

Versatility: Infusions can be made with a single herb or a blend, allowing for customization based on therapeutic needs or flavour preferences. This versatility makes them a favourite in herbal medicine, catering to various health goals and taste profiles.
Example: A blend of peppermint and licorice root can be used for digestive support and a pleasant, sweet flavour.

Tea
Tea: Traditionally refers to the leaves of the Camellia sinensis plant, but in herbal medicine, 'tea' often refers to a light infusion of various herbs.
Process: Herbal teas are brewed in a similar manner to infusions but are often steeped for a shorter time. This balance caters to both therapeutic benefits and a pleasant drinking experience.
Example: A cup of peppermint tea is typically steeped for about 5 minutes, providing a refreshing and mildly therapeutic beverage.

Varieties: There are many varieties of herbal teas, each with unique flavour profiles and health benefits. This diversity allows for endless exploration and enjoyment of different herbal properties.
Example: Ginger tea, known for its spicy flavour, is commonly used to soothe nausea and improve digestion.

Benefits of Teas
Antioxidants: Many herbal teas are rich in antioxidants, which help combat oxidative stress and inflammation. Regular consumption of antioxidant-rich teas supports overall health and longevity.
Example: Rooibos tea, high in antioxidants, is popular for its health benefits and sweet, nutty flavour.

Digestive Health: Certain teas, like peppermint or ginger, are known for their ability to aid digestion. These teas can soothe an upset stomach, relieve bloating, and improve overall digestive function.
Example: After a heavy meal, a cup of ginger tea can help settle the stomach and promote digestion.

Relaxation: Herbs like chamomile are renowned for their calming effects and are often consumed before bed to promote sleep. These teas help reduce anxiety and stress, supporting mental well-being. -
Example: A warm cup of chamomile tea before

bedtime can enhance relaxation and improve sleep quality.

Cultural Significance
Global Tradition: The practice of making infusions and teas is a global tradition, with each culture having its own preferred herbs and methods of preparation.
Examples:
China: Green tea has been enjoyed for centuries, celebrated for its health benefits and cultural significance.
South America: Yerba mate is a social drink shared among friends, fostering a sense of community. -
Europe: Herbal infusions like chamomile and peppermint have long been used for their medicinal properties.
Social Aspect: Sharing a cup of herbal tea is a social ritual in many societies, fostering a sense of community and well-being. In many cultures, tea ceremonies and rituals are important social activities that bring people together. These practices often include specific etiquette and traditions that enhance the experience and cultural connection. In Japan, the tea ceremony (Chanoyu) is a cultural practice that emphasises mindfulness and respect.

Modern Applications:

Health and Wellness Industry: Infusions and teas have seen a resurgence in popularity within the health and wellness industry, with many brands offering a wide range of herbal blends for various health concerns.

Trends: There is a growing demand for natural and holistic health solutions, driving the popularity of herbal teas. Many companies now offer specialised blends targeting specific health issues, such as detox teas, sleep aids, and immune boosters.
Example: Detox teas with ingredients like dandelion and burdock root are marketed for their cleansing properties.

Convenience: Modern life has introduced tea bags and ready-to-drink herbal infusions, making it easier than ever to enjoy the benefits of herbal medicine. - **Examples:** Tea bags provide a convenient and mess-free way to brew herbal teas, suitable for busy lifestyles. Ready-to-drink options are available in stores, offering herbal infusions that can be consumed on the go. Bottled iced herbal teas like hibiscus or green tea provide a refreshing and healthy alternative to sugary beverages.

Safety Considerations: Quality of Herbs Always use high-quality, organic herbs to avoid contaminants like pesticides and ensure the safety and efficacy of your herbal remedies.

Practical Tips: Purchase herbs from reputable suppliers who provide certification of purity and quality. Check for organic certification to ensure that the herbs are free from harmful chemicals. If growing your own herbs, use organic farming practices and avoid chemical pesticides.

Example: Organic chamomile flowers from a trusted supplier ensure you get a pure and safe product.

Medical Conditions: Some herbs can interact with medications or may not be suitable for people with certain medical conditions.

Practical Tips: Discuss your current medications and health conditions with your healthcare provider to identify any potential interactions. Start with small doses of new herbs to monitor for any adverse reactions. Be aware of the specific contraindications of each herb, especially if you have chronic health conditions.

Example: St. John's Wort can interact with antidepressants and should be used cautiously.

Tinctures and Extracts

Tinctures and extracts are concentrated herbal preparations that capture the essential properties of plants. They are commonly used in natural medicine to provide the therapeutic benefits of herbs in a potent and easily consumable form.

Tinctures: are typically made by soaking herbs in a solvent such as alcohol, glycerin, or vinegar. This process extracts the active constituents of the herbs into the liquid, which is then strained and bottled. Tinctures are highly concentrated and only require small dosages.

Extracts: can be made using similar processes, but they encompass a broader range of preparation methods. They can include not just liquid extracts (like tinctures) but also solid and semi-solid forms such as powdered extracts and pastes.

Preparation Methods

1. **Alcohol-Based Tinctures:** Alcohol-based tinctures are herbal extracts made by infusing herbs in alcohol, typically vodka or brandy, to create a potent and long-lasting medicinal remedy. Here's a detailed explanation of the ingredients and process involved in making alcohol-based tinctures.

Ingredients:
1. Fresh or dried herbs: Choose herbs with known medicinal properties, such as echinacea, chamomile, or peppermint. Ensure that the herbs are of high quality and free from pesticides or contaminants.
2. Alcohol: Use alcohol with a high proof (40-60% or 80-120 proof), as it acts as a potent solvent to extract the beneficial compounds from the herbs. Vodka or brandy is commonly used for tinctures.
3. A jar: Opt for a glass jar with a tight-fitting lid to prevent evaporation of alcohol during the steeping process.

Process:
1. Chop the herbs: Finely chop or grind the herbs to increase their surface area and promote better extraction. 2. Place herbs in a jar: Fill the jar about 1/3 to 1/2 full with the chopped herbs.
3. Cover with alcohol: Pour the alcohol over the herbs, ensuring they are completely submerged. The ratio of herbs to alcohol is typically 1 part herbs to 3-5 parts alcohol, depending on the desired potency. **4. Seal the jar:** Close the lid tightly to prevent evaporation and contamination.
5. Steep the herbs: Store the jar in a dark, cool place for 4-6 weeks, shaking it daily to encourage the extraction process.

6. Strain the liquid: After the steeping period, strain the liquid through a cheesecloth or a fine mesh strainer.

7. Bottle the tincture: Transfer the tincture to a dark glass bottle, label it with the name of the herb and the date, and store it in a cool, dark place. Alcohol-based tinctures can be used as natural remedies for various ailments, such as reducing inflammation, relieving stress, or promoting sleep. It's important to note that while tinctures are generally safe, always consult with a healthcare provider before using them, especially if you have any medical conditions or take prescription medications.

1. Chop the herbs finely to increase the surface area.
2. Place the herbs in a jar and cover them with alcohol. The alcohol should be at least 40-60% (80-120 proof).
3. Seal the jar tightly and store it in a dark, cool place for 4-6 weeks, shaking it daily.
4. After the steeping period, strain the liquid through a cheesecloth or a fine mesh strainer, squeezing out as much liquid as possible from the herbs.
5. Store the tincture in a dark glass bottle, label it with the name and date, and keep it in a cool, dark place.

2.. Glycerin-Based Tinctures (Glycerites): Glycerin-based tinctures, also known as glycerites, are herbal extracts made using vegetable glycerin instead of alcohol. These tinctures are suitable for individuals who prefer to avoid alcohol or for children. Here's a detailed explanation of the ingredients and process involved in making glycerin-based tinctures:

Ingredients:
1. Herbs: Select fresh or dried herbs with known medicinal properties. Ensure the herbs are clean and free from contaminants.
2. Vegetable glycerin: A plant-based, sweet-tasting liquid used as a solvent to extract the beneficial compounds from herbs.
3. Water: Used to dilute the glycerin and help with the extraction process.

Process:
1. Mix glycerin and water: Combine three parts glycerin with one part water in a bowl. Stir well to create a homogenous mixture.
2. Follow the same procedure as alcohol-based tinctures: Place chopped herbs in a glass jar, cover them with the glycerin-water mixture, and seal the jar tightly.
3. Steep the herbs: Store the jar in a dark, cool place for 4-6 weeks, shaking it daily to promote the extraction process.
4. Strain the liquid: After the steeping period, strain the liquid through a cheesecloth or fine mesh

strainer, squeezing out as much liquid as possible from the herbs.

5. Bottle the glycerite: Transfer the glycerite to a dark glass bottle, label it with the name of the herb and the date, and store it in a cool, dark place. Glycerites are a good alternative for individuals who are sensitive to alcohol or prefer a more palatable taste. They can be used for the same medicinal purposes as alcohol-based tinctures, such as reducing inflammation, relieving stress, or promoting sleep. However, always consult with a healthcare provider before using any herbal remedy to ensure it is safe and appropriate for your specific needs.

Ingredients: Herbs, vegetable glycerin, and water.
Process:
1. Combine three parts glycerin with one part water.
2. Follow the same procedure as for alcohol-based tinctures, substituting the glycerin-water mixture for alcohol.
3. Glycerites are a good alternative for children or individuals avoiding alcohol.

3. Vinegar-Based Tinctures: Vinegar-based tinctures are another type of herbal extract made using apple cider vinegar instead of alcohol. They offer an alternative method of extraction and are suitable for individuals who prefer to avoid alcohol or glycerin-based tinctures. Here's a detailed explanation of the ingredients and process involved in making vinegar-based tinctures:

Ingredients:
1. **Herbs:** Choose fresh or dried herbs with known medicinal properties. Make sure the herbs are clean and free from contaminants.
2. **Apple cider vinegar:** A fermented, acidic liquid made from apple juice that acts as a solvent to extract the beneficial compounds from herbs.

Process:
1. **Fill a jar with herbs:** Place chopped herbs in a glass jar, filling it about 1/3 to 1/2 full.
2. **Cover with apple cider vinegar:** Pour the vinegar over the herbs, ensuring they are completely submerged. The ratio of herbs to vinegar is typically 1 part herbs to 3-5 parts vinegar, depending on the desired potency.
3. **Use a non-corrosive lid:** Since vinegar can react with metal, it's essential to use a plastic lid or a layer of parchment paper between the jar and a metal lid to prevent corrosion.
4. **Steep the herbs:** Store the jar in a dark, cool place for 4-6 weeks, shaking it daily to promote the extraction process.
5. **Strain the liquid:** After the steeping period, strain the liquid through a cheesecloth or a fine mesh

strainer, squeezing out as much liquid as possible from the herbs.

6. Bottle the tincture: Transfer the vinegar-based tincture to a dark glass bottle, label it with the name of the herb and the date, and store it in a cool, dark place. Vinegar-based tinctures can be used for the same medicinal purposes as alcohol or glycerin-based tinctures, such as reducing inflammation, relieving stress, or promoting sleep. However, always consult with a healthcare provider before using any herbal remedy to ensure it is safe and appropriate for your specific needs.

Ingredients:
Herbs and apple cider vinegar.

Process:
1. Fill a jar with herbs and cover with apple cider vinegar.
2. Proceed as with alcohol tinctures, but be sure to use a plastic lid or a layer of parchment paper between the jar and a metal lid to prevent corrosion from the vinegar.

4. Powdered Extracts: Powdered extracts are a concentrated form of herbal medicine made by drying and grinding herbs into a fine powder. This method allows for easy encapsulation or the creation of tablets, making it convenient for consumption. Here's a detailed explanation of the ingredients and process involved in making powdered extracts.

Ingredients:
1. **Herbs:** Choose fresh or dried herbs with known medicinal properties. Make sure the herbs are clean and free from contaminants.
2. **Drying agent (optional):** Some herbalists use a drying agent like silica gel or calcium chloride to speed up the drying process.

Process:
1. **Dry the herbs:** Spread the herbs on a clean, dry surface, or use a dehydrator to dry them thoroughly. This step is crucial to prevent mold growth during storage.
2. **Grind the herbs:** Once the herbs are completely dry, grind them into a fine powder using a mortar and pestle, spice grinder, or a food processor.
3. **Encapsulate or create tablets:** You can encapsulate the powdered extract using empty capsules or compress it into tablets. Alternatively, you can mix the powder with a small amount of water or honey to consume it directly.
4. **Store the powdered extract:** Keep the powdered extract in an airtight container, away from heat, light, and moisture. Powdered extracts offer a convenient way to consume herbs and can be tailored to individual dosage requirements. However, always consult with a healthcare provider before using any herbal remedy to ensure it is safe and appropriate for your specific needs.

Ingredients: Herbs and a drying agent.
Process:
1. Herbs are dried and ground into a fine powder.
2. The powder can be encapsulated or used to make tablets.

5. Fluid Extracts: Fluid extracts are potent herbal preparations that are similar to tinctures but are more concentrated due to a higher herb-to-solvent ratio. They are made using a combination of alcohol and water as solvents. This method extracts and preserves the medicinal properties of herbs effectively. Here's a detailed explanation of the ingredients and process involved in making fluid extracts.

Ingredients:
1. **Herbs:** Select fresh or dried herbs with known medicinal properties. Ensure that the herbs are of high quality and free from pesticides or contaminants.
2. **Alcohol:** Use high-proof alcohol (40-60% or 80-120 proof) to effectively extract the beneficial compounds from the herbs.
3. **Water:** Use distilled or purified water to reduce the risk of contamination and maintain the purity of the extract.

Process:

1. Determine the herb-to-solvent ratio: Fluid extracts typically have a higher herb-to-solvent ratio than tinctures, often 1:1 or 1:2 (one part herb to one or two parts solvent).

2. Combine ingredients: Place the herbs in a glass jar, and cover them with the alcohol and water mixture, following your chosen ratio.

3. Seal the jar: Close the lid tightly to prevent evaporation and contamination.

4. Macerate the herbs: Store the jar in a dark, cool place for 4-6 weeks, shaking it daily to encourage the extraction process.

5. Decant the liquid: After the maceration period, strain the liquid through a cheesecloth or a fine mesh strainer, squeezing out as much liquid as possible from the herbs. Reserve the liquid.

6. Reserve the marc: Retain the marc (the spent herbal material) for further processing.

7. Concentrate the liquid (optional): Reduce the volume of the liquid by evaporating the alcohol and water using gentle heat in a well-ventilated area. This step is optional and depends on the desired final concentration.

8. Combine the concentrated liquid with the reserved marc: Allow the concentrated liquid to reabsorb into the marc for at least one week, then strain and bottle it. Fluid extracts are highly concentrated, and dosages may need to be adjusted accordingly. Always consult with a healthcare

provider before using any herbal remedy to ensure it is safe and appropriate for your specific needs.
Ingredients: Herbs, alcohol, and water.
Process:
1. Similar to tinctures but more concentrated.
2. The ratio of herb to solvent is higher, often 1:1 or 1:2.

Tinctures and Extracts: An In-Depth Guide

Tinctures and extracts are concentrated herbal preparations that use solvents to extract and preserve the medicinal properties of plants. These potent remedies have been used for centuries in traditional medicine systems worldwide, offering an effective way to harness the healing power of nature.

Benefits of Tinctures and Extracts

1. Potency: Tinctures and extracts are prepared by extracting and concentrating the active compounds of an herb or plant in a solvent, such as alcohol, glycerin, or vinegar. The resulting solution is highly concentrated, containing a higher amount of active compounds compared to the original plant material. This makes them effective even in small doses. - Alcohol and glycerin are excellent solvents, as they can extract a wide range of compounds, such as alkaloids, flavonoids, and terpenoids, which are responsible for the therapeutic effects of the plant.

2. Long Shelf Life: Alcohol-based tinctures have a long shelf life, often lasting several years, as alcohol acts as a preservative, preventing bacterial and fungal growth. Glycerin and vinegar tinctures, although not as effective as alcohol in preserving the extract, still offer an extended shelf life compared to fresh herbs or other plant preparations.

3. Convenience: Tinctures are easy to administer and can be taken in various ways, such as directly under the tongue (sublingually), added to water or tea, or even applied topically, depending on the intended use. The dropper that comes with most tincture bottles allows for accurate and consistent dosing, enabling users to control the amount they consume.

4. Bioavailability: The liquid form of tinctures allows for quick absorption into the bloodstream, as they do not need to be broken down like solid forms of medication. This results in faster therapeutic effects. Alcohol, specifically, enhances the bioavailability of certain compounds by increasing their solubility and absorption in the body. This makes tinctures prepared with alcohol-based solvents more effective in delivering the desired therapeutic effects. These factors contribute to the overall effectiveness, convenience, and appeal of using tinctures and extracts as herbal remedies or supplements. Tinctures and extracts are highly concentrated, making them powerful and effective even in small doses.

Common Uses and Applications

1. Immune Support: Echinacea tinctures are known to stimulate the immune system, helping to fight off colds and flu more effectively. Elderberry tinctures are popular for their antiviral properties, which can aid in preventing and shortening the duration of respiratory illnesses.

2. Digestive Health: Peppermint tinctures can provide relief from digestive issues like bloating, indigestion, and stomach discomfort by relaxing the muscles in the digestive tract. Ginger tinctures are effective at easing nausea, vomiting, and other digestive problems due to their anti-inflammatory and antiemetic properties.

3. Stress and Anxiety: Valerian root tinctures have sedative properties that can help alleviate anxiety and promote relaxation. Chamomile tinctures are well-known for their calming effects, which can soothe the nerves and encourage relaxation.

4. Pain Relief: Willow bark tinctures contain salicin, a compound similar to aspirin, and are used for pain relief and reducing inflammation. Turmeric tinctures are potent anti-inflammatories, making them useful in managing pain associated with arthritis and other inflammatory conditions.

5. Sleep Aid: Passionflower tinctures have calming effects on the nervous system, which can help improve sleep quality and promote relaxation. Valerian tinctures, as mentioned earlier, are often used for their sedative properties that can aid in sleep.

Safety and Considerations

1. Quality of Ingredients: Opt for high-quality, organic herbs to ensure that your tinctures are free from pesticides, herbicides, and other harmful chemicals. Using fresh, high-quality ingredients improves the overall effectiveness and potency of the final product.

2. Proper Dosage: Follow recommended dosages on the product label or consult a healthcare professional to determine the appropriate amount for your specific needs. Dosage may vary based on factors such as age, weight, and health conditions. Exceeding recommended dosages can increase the risk of adverse effects or reduced efficacy.

3. Alcohol Sensitivity: If you are sensitive to alcohol, consider using glycerin or vinegar-based tinctures instead. Alcohol-based tinctures may contain up to 60-70% alcohol, which can cause side effects in sensitive individuals.

4. Interactions and Contraindications: Be aware that some herbs may interact with prescription medications or worsen existing health conditions. Consult with a healthcare professional before using tinctures, especially if you are pregnant or breastfeeding, have a pre-existing health condition, or are taking medication.

5. Storage: Proper storage is essential to maintain the potency and shelf life of your tinctures. Store tinctures in dark glass bottles, away from direct heat and sunlight. Keep bottles tightly sealed and store in a cool, dry place.

Salves and Balms

Salves and balms are topical preparations used to soothe, heal, and protect the skin. They are made by infusing herbs into a carrier oil, then thickening the mixture with beeswax or other natural waxes to create a semi-solid consistency. Both terms are often used interchangeably, though "balms" may sometimes refer to a firmer product.

Ingredients

1. Herbs: Healing Herbs help soothe and repair damaged skin, promoting faster healing. Examples include calendula, comfrey, plantain, and yarrow.
Anti-inflammatory Herbs: reduce inflammation and can ease pain. Arnica, St. John's Wort, and chamomile are commonly used.
Antimicrobial Herbs: inhibit the growth of bacteria, fungi, and viruses. Tea tree, lavender, and thyme are popular choices.
Skin-Nourishing Herbs: offer essential nutrients to the skin, promoting its overall health. Lavender, rosemary, and rose petals are great options.

2. Carrier Oils: Common Oils serve as the base for most herbal salves and tinctures, diluting essential oils and carrying nutrients into the skin. Olive oil, coconut oil, jojoba oil, and almond oil are frequently used.
Specialty Oils: offer unique therapeutic benefits and can enhance the effectiveness of the final product. Examples include tamanu oil, rosehip seed oil, and calendula-infused oil.

3. Waxes: Beeswax is the most commonly used thickening agent in herbal salves, providing texture and solidifying the mixture.
Vegan Alternatives: such as candelilla wax and carnauba wax can replace beeswax for those following a plant-based lifestyle.

4. Essential Oils: Essential oils provide additional therapeutic benefits and pleasant aromas to herbal concoctions. Popular choices include lavender, tea tree, peppermint, and eucalyptus.

5. Optional Ingredients: Butters like shea butter and cocoa butter add extra moisturising properties to herbal salves.

Vitamins: such as vitamin E oil serve as natural preservatives and provide additional skin nutrients.

Preparation Methods
1. Infusing the Oil, Cold Infusion: Fill a jar with dried herbs and cover with carrier oil. - Seal and place in a sunny spot for 4-6 weeks, shaking daily. - Strain the oil through cheesecloth, squeezing out all the liquid from the herbs.

Hot Infusion: Combine herbs and oil in a double boiler or slow cooker. Heat on low for several hours, ensuring the oil does not get too hot (under 110°F). - Strain as above.

2. Making the Salve/Balm, Ingredients: Infused oil, beeswax (or alternative), essential oils (optional).

Process
1. Measure ingredients: Measure out your chosen infused oil and wax using the desired ratio. A common ratio for a medium-firm salve is 1 cup of

infused oil to 1 ounce of beeswax (or vegan alternative). Adjust the ratio as needed for a firmer or softer consistency.

2. Set up a double boiler: Fill a saucepan with a few inches of water, ensuring the water doesn't touch the bottom of the bowl or glass container you'll use for melting the ingredients. Place the glass container or bowl on top of the saucepan.

3. Heat the oil and wax: Add the measured infused oil and wax to the glass container or bowl in the double boiler. Heat the water in the saucepan over medium heat until the wax melts completely. Stir occasionally to ensure the wax and oil combine evenly.

4. Remove from heat and add essential oils: Once the wax has melted and the mixture is well-combined, carefully remove the glass container or bowl from the heat. Allow it to cool slightly before adding essential oils, if desired. Add 10-20 drops of essential oil per cup of infused oil and stir well.

5. Pour into containers: Pour the mixture into clean, sterilised jars or tins. To sterilise containers, boil them in water for 10 minutes or wash them with hot, soapy water and dry them in an oven at 250°F (120°C) for 15 minutes.

6. Cool and solidify: Allow the salve or balm to cool and solidify completely before sealing the containers. This can take several hours at room temperature or about an hour in the refrigerator.

Once cooled, the consistency should be firm yet easily spreadable. Your homemade herbal salve or balm is now ready to use! Apply it to the affected area as needed, and remember to perform a patch test before applying it to larger areas of the skin.

Benefits of Salves and Balms
1. Localised Treatment: Directly apply to the affected area, ensuring targeted treatment. Ideal for skin issues such as cuts, scrapes, burns, insect bites, and rashes.
2. Skin Protection: Forms a protective barrier on the skin, locking in moisture and shielding from environmental irritants. Beeswax and other waxes provide a breathable barrier without clogging pores.
3. Natural Ingredients: Made from natural, often organic ingredients, reducing the risk of adverse reactions compared to synthetic products. Free from preservatives, parabens, and artificial fragrances.
4. Versatility: Can be customised for various uses: healing salves, moisturising balms, lip balms, muscle rubs, and more. Essential oils can be added for additional benefits, such as anti-inflammatory, antiseptic, or calming effects.

Common Uses and Applications
1. Healing Salves, Ingredients: Calendula, comfrey, plantain, beeswax, lavender essential oil.

Uses: Promote healing of minor cuts, scrapes, and burns; soothe rashes and insect bites.

2. Muscle and Joint Balms, Ingredients: Arnica, St. John's Wort, cayenne pepper, beeswax, peppermint and eucalyptus essential oils.

Uses: Relieve muscle soreness, joint pain, and inflammation.

3. Moisturizing Balms, Ingredients: Shea butter, cocoa butter, olive oil, beeswax, rose and chamomile essential oils.

Uses: Deeply moisturise dry, cracked skin; soothe eczema and dermatitis.

4. Lip Balms, Ingredients: Coconut oil, beeswax, shea butter, peppermint essential oil.

Uses: Hydrate and protect lips while preventing chapping and cracking with these lip balms.

5. Antiseptic Balms, Ingredients: Tea tree oil, thyme, lavender, beeswax.

Uses: Treat minor infections, prevent bacterial growth, soothe skin irritations.

Safety and Considerations

1. Patch Test: Always perform a patch test before using a new salve or balm to ensure there is no allergic reaction. Apply a small amount to the inner forearm and wait 24 hours for any signs of irritation.

2. Storage: Store in a cool, dark place to prevent the oils from going rancid. Properly stored salves and balms can last up to a year or more.

3. Quality of Ingredients: Use high-quality, organic ingredients whenever possible to maximise the therapeutic benefits and minimise contaminants. - Ensure the herbs are properly dried to prevent mould and bacteria growth during infusion.

4. Proper Hygiene: Use clean, sterilised equipment and containers to avoid contamination. Wash hands thoroughly before handling the finished product.

5. Consultation with a Healthcare Professional: Consult a healthcare professional before using herbal salves and balms, especially if you have existing health conditions or are taking medications. Some herbs and essential oils may interact with certain medications or exacerbate specific health conditions.

Essential Oils and Aromatherapy

Essential oils are concentrated, volatile plant extracts obtained through various methods such as steam distillation, cold pressing, or solvent extraction. These oils capture the essence, aroma, and therapeutic properties of the plant, containing a wide range of beneficial compounds.

Extraction Methods

1. Steam Distillation: Steam is passed through plant material, vaporising volatile compounds. Vapour then condenses, separating essential oil from water, preserving delicate plant components.

Process: Plant material is placed in a distillation apparatus, and steam is passed through the plant material, vaporising the volatile compounds.
Commonly Used For: Lavender, eucalyptus, peppermint, tea tree.

2. Cold Pressing: Used primarily for citrus oils, this method mechanically presses the plant material (usually the peels) to release the oils. This process is also known as expression.
Commonly Used For: Lemon, orange, grapefruit, lime.

3. Solvent Extraction: A solvent (usually hexane or ethanol) is used to dissolve the essential oils from the plant material. After the solvent is removed, a concentrated form of essential oil called an absolute is left.
Commonly Used For: Jasmine, rose, vanilla.

4. CO_2 Extraction: Carbon dioxide is used under high pressure and variable temperatures to extract the oils. This method preserves more of the plant's natural compounds and is considered a superior extraction technique.
Commonly Used For: Frankincense, chamomile, ginger.

Benefits and Uses of Essential Oils
1. Aromatherapy: Aromatherapy is the practice of using essential oils for therapeutic benefits through inhalation or topical application.

Mechanism: When inhaled, essential oils interact with the olfactory system and limbic system in the brain, influencing emotions, memory, and hormonal responses.

2. Common Essential Oils and Their Benefits:

1. Lavender: Lavender essential oil is known for its calming and soothing properties, which can help promote relaxation and sleep. It's also helpful in relieving skin irritations due to its anti-inflammatory properties.

2. Peppermint: Peppermint essential oil has an energising effect and can help relieve headaches and aid digestion. Additionally, it can help clear respiratory passages due to its cooling and refreshing properties.

3. Tea Tree: Tea tree essential oil is highly valued for its antimicrobial, antifungal, and antiseptic properties. It's commonly used to treat skin infections and wounds.

4. Eucalyptus: Eucalyptus essential oil is known for its decongestant properties, making it useful for respiratory support and clearing the airways. It's also helpful for relieving muscle pain.

5. Lemon: Lemon essential oil has uplifting and detoxifying properties, which can help cleanse and purify the air. It's often used to promote a refreshing and invigorating atmosphere.

6. Chamomile: Chamomile essential oil has calming properties that can help promote restful sleep and reduce inflammation. It's also gentle on the skin and can be used to soothe irritated or sensitive skin.

Aromatherapy Techniques
1. Diffusion, Devices: Ultrasonic diffusers, nebulizers, and passive diffusers.
Benefits: Disperses essential oils into the air, providing continuous inhalation benefits.
2. Steam Inhalation, Method: Add a few drops of essential oil to a bowl of hot water, cover the head with a towel, and inhale the steam.
Benefits: Effective for respiratory issues, colds, and congestion.
3. Topical Application Method: Dilute essential oils in a carrier oil and apply to the skin.
Benefits: Localised treatment for pain, skin conditions, and relaxation.
4. Bath Method: Add a few drops of essential oil to a carrier oil or Epsom salts, then add to bathwater.
Benefits: Full-body relaxation, skin nourishment, and stress relief.
5. Compresses, Method: Add essential oils to hot or cold water, soak a cloth, and apply to the affected area.
Benefits: Pain relief, inflammation reduction, and muscle relaxation It's important to note that essential oils should always be used with caution and proper dilution to avoid any potential skin irritation or adverse reactions. Consulting a professional

aromatherapist or healthcare provider is recommended before incorporating essential oils into your daily routine.

Safety and Considerations
1. Dilution Ratios, Adults: Typically, a 2-3% dilution (10-15 drops of essential oil per ounce of carrier oil) is safe for most topical applications. **Children:** Use a lower dilution (1% or less), and avoid certain oils like peppermint and eucalyptus.
2. Skin Sensitivity: Always perform a patch test before using a new essential oil topically. Apply a diluted oil to a small area of skin and wait 24 hours to check for reactions.
3. Quality of Oils: Use high-quality, pure essential oils from reputable sources. Look for oils labelled as "100% pure" and avoid those with synthetic additives.Quality of Oils.
4. Storage: Store essential oils in dark glass bottles, away from heat and light, to preserve their potency and shelf life.
5. Contraindications and Interactions: Certain essential oils can interact with medications or exacerbate medical conditions. Consult with a healthcare provider if you have any health concerns or are pregnant, breastfeeding, or have underlying medical conditions.

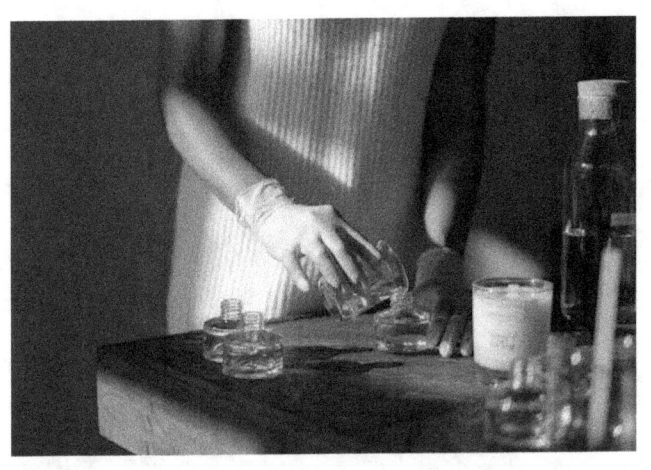

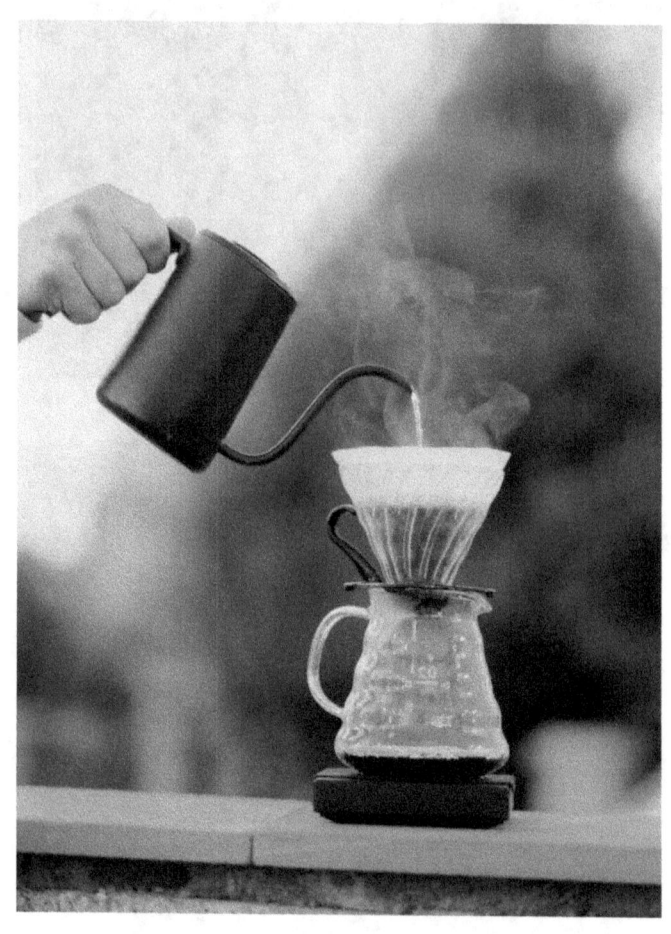

Chapter 3: Common Herbs and Their Uses

Medicinal Properties of Herbs

Herbal medicine, also known as phytotherapy or botanical medicine, utilises plants and plant extracts for medicinal purposes. Herbs have been used for thousands of years across different cultures for their therapeutic properties. They contain a wide array of bioactive compounds, including alkaloids, flavonoids, terpenes, and phenolic compounds, which contribute to their medicinal effects.

Common Medicinal Properties of Herbs

1. Anti-inflammatory: Herbs with anti-inflammatory properties reduce inflammation in the body, alleviating pain and swelling. Examples include turmeric, ginger, and boswellia.

2. Antioxidant: Antioxidant herbs neutralise free radicals in the body, protecting cells from oxidative damage and reducing the risk of chronic diseases. Examples include green tea, rosemary, and oregano.

3. Antimicrobial: Antimicrobial herbs inhibit the growth of microorganisms such as bacteria, viruses, fungi, and parasites, helping to prevent and treat infections. Examples include garlic, thyme, and tea tree oil.

4. **Adaptogenic:** Adaptogenic herbs help the body adapt to stressors, promoting resilience and overall well-being. They balance the body's stress response system and support adrenal function. Examples include ashwagandha, rhodiola, and holy basil.

5. **Sedative/Anxiolytic:** Sedative and anxiolytic herbs have calming and relaxing effects on the nervous system, reducing anxiety, promoting sleep, and relieving tension. Examples include chamomile, valerian, and passionflower.

6. **Digestive:** Digestive herbs support healthy digestion and alleviate digestive discomforts such as indigestion, bloating, and nausea. They may stimulate digestion, reduce inflammation, and promote gut health. Examples include peppermint, ginger, and fennel.

7. **Hepatoprotective:** Hepatoprotective herbs protect the liver from damage and support its detoxification functions. They may help prevent liver diseases and improve liver function. Examples include milk thistle, dandelion, and artichoke.

8. Immunomodulatory: Immunomodulatory herbs regulate the immune system, enhancing immune function and helping the body fight infections and diseases. They may stimulate immune activity or modulate immune responses. Examples include echinacea, astragalus, and reishi mushroom.

9. Cardioprotective: Cardioprotective herbs support heart health and reduce the risk of cardiovascular diseases. They may lower blood pressure, cholesterol levels, and inflammation, improving overall cardiovascular function. Examples include hawthorn, garlic, and cayenne.

10. Analgesic: Analgesic herbs relieve pain by reducing the perception of pain signals in the body. They may act as mild to moderate pain relievers for various conditions. Examples include white willow bark, cayenne, and arnica.

Modes of Administration
1. Teas and Infusions: Herbs can be brewed into teas or infusions by steeping them in hot water. This method extracts the active constituents, making them suitable for internal use.

2. Tinctures and Extracts: Tinctures and extracts are concentrated herbal preparations made by extracting the active compounds from herbs using alcohol, glycerin, or vinegar. They are often taken orally and provide a potent and convenient way to consume herbs.

3. Topical Applications: Herbs can be applied topically in various forms such as creams, ointments, salves, and poultices. This allows for localised treatment of skin conditions, wounds, and muscle pain.

4. Capsules and Tablets: Herbs are encapsulated or compressed into tablets for convenient oral consumption. This method provides a standardised dosage and is suitable for herbs with a bitter taste or strong odour.

5. Inhalation: Inhalation of herbal vapours or essential oils is used in aromatherapy to provide respiratory and emotional benefits. This method can be achieved through steam inhalation, diffusers, or aromatic sprays.

Safety and Considerations
1. High-Quality and Pure Herbs for Optimal Safety and Effectiveness: It's important to prioritise quality and purity when using herbs, ensuring they are sourced from reliable suppliers and free from harmful contaminants. This can ensure optimal safety and effectiveness in your wellness routine.

2. Dosage and Administration: Follow recommended dosage guidelines and administration methods for each herb. Some herbs may be toxic in large doses or when used improperly.

3. Potential Interactions: Be aware of potential herb-drug interactions, especially if you are taking medications or have underlying health conditions. Consult with a healthcare professional before using herbs, especially if you are pregnant, breastfeeding, or have medical concerns.

4. Identifying and Managing Allergies and Sensitivities: Be aware of potential allergic reactions or sensitivities to herbs. To avoid adverse effects, perform a patch test or use small doses initially to check for tolerance. If any allergic symptoms occur, discontinue use immediately and consult a healthcare professional.

5. Storage and Shelf Life: Store dried herbs in a cool, dry place away from direct sunlight to preserve their potency and extend their shelf life. Properly stored herbs can maintain their efficacy for several months to a few years.

Culinary Herbs with Health Benefits

Herbs have long been utilised to support and enhance digestive health due to their natural properties, including anti-inflammatory, carminative, and soothing effects on the gastrointestinal tract. Incorporating these herbs into your diet and lifestyle can promote digestion, alleviate discomfort, and support overall gastrointestinal well-being.

Common Herbs for Digestive Health
1. Peppermint (Mentha piperita): Peppermint contains menthol, which has antispasmodic properties that help relax the muscles of the digestive tract. It also soothes digestive discomfort and reduces bloating and gas.
Uses: Peppermint tea is commonly used to relieve indigestion, gas, and bloating. It may also help alleviate symptoms of irritable bowel syndrome (IBS) and promote bile flow.

2. Ginger (Zingiber officinale): Ginger contains gingerol, a bioactive compound with anti-inflammatory and carminative properties. It stimulates digestion, relieves nausea, and reduces intestinal cramping and gas.
Uses: Ginger tea or fresh ginger root can be consumed to alleviate nausea, indigestion, and

motion sickness. It may also help reduce symptoms of gastrointestinal upset.

3. Chamomile (Matricaria chamomilla): Chamomile has anti-inflammatory, antispasmodic, and calming effects on the digestive system. It helps soothe the stomach, reduce acidity, and alleviate digestive discomfort.
Uses: Chamomile tea is often consumed to relieve indigestion, bloating, and abdominal cramps. It may also promote relaxation and reduce stress-related digestive issues.

4. Fennel (Foeniculum vulgare): Fennel contains volatile oils like anethole, which have carminative and anti-inflammatory properties. It helps relax the gastrointestinal muscles, reduce gas, and alleviate bloating and indigestion.
Uses: Fennel tea or seeds can be consumed after meals to aid digestion and relieve gas and bloating. It may also help stimulate appetite and promote healthy bowel movements.

5. Dandelion (Taraxacum officinale): Dandelion root has bitter compounds that stimulate digestive juices, including bile production, which aids in the digestion of fats. It also has diuretic properties that help eliminate toxins from the body.

Uses: Dandelion root tea or supplements can be consumed to support liver and gallbladder health, improve digestion, and relieve constipation.

6. **Licorice Root (Glycyrrhiza glabra):** Licorice root contains glycyrrhizin, which has demulcent and anti-inflammatory properties that soothe and protect the mucous membranes of the digestive tract. It also supports healthy stomach acid production.
Uses: Licorice root tea or supplements are used to relieve symptoms of heartburn, acid reflux, and gastritis. It may also help soothe throat irritation and promote ulcer healing.

7. **Turmeric (Curcuma longa):** Turmeric contains curcumin, a bioactive compound with anti-inflammatory and antioxidant properties. It helps reduce inflammation in the digestive tract, improve digestion, and protect against gastrointestinal diseases.
Uses: Turmeric can be added to curries, soups, and smoothies to promote digestive health. Turmeric supplements may also be taken to support overall gastrointestinal function.

Incorporating Herbs for Digestive Health into Your Routine
1. **Herbal Teas:** Brew digestive herbs like peppermint, ginger, chamomile, or fennel into teas

and sip them before or after meals to aid digestion and relieve discomfort.

2. Herbal Supplements: Take herbal supplements containing digestive herbs in capsule or tablet form to support gastrointestinal health. Choose high-quality products from reputable brands.

3. Culinary Use: Incorporate digestive herbs like ginger, turmeric, and fennel into your cooking. Use them in soups, stews, stir-fries, or marinades to enhance flavour and promote digestion.

4. Tinctures and Extracts: Add digestive herb tinctures or extracts to water or juice and consume them before meals to stimulate digestion and reduce bloating and gas.

5. Topical Applications: Some digestive herbs can be applied topically to alleviate digestive discomfort. For example, peppermint oil can be diluted and massaged onto the abdomen to relieve gas and bloating.

Safety and Considerations
1. Quality and Purity: Choose high-quality, organic herbs from reputable sources to ensure purity and potency. Avoid herbs that may be contaminated with pesticides, heavy metals, or other toxins.

2. Dosage and Administration: Follow recommended dosage guidelines for each herb and consult with a healthcare professional if you have any concerns or medical conditions.

3. Pregnancy and Medical Conditions: Some herbs may not be suitable for pregnant or breastfeeding women or individuals with certain medical conditions. Consult with a healthcare provider before using herbal remedies, especially if you are taking medications or have underlying health concerns.

4. Allergies and Sensitivities: Be aware of potential allergies or sensitivities to certain herbs. Monitor for any adverse reactions and discontinue use if you experience any symptoms.

5. Moderation: While herbs are generally safe for consumption in food amounts, excessive intake or prolonged use of certain herbs may cause gastrointestinal discomfort. As with any dietary supplement, use herbs for digestive health in moderation and listen to your body's response.

Herbs for Immune Support

Herbs have been used for centuries to support and strengthen the immune system. Packed with vitamins, minerals, antioxidants, and other bioactive compounds, certain herbs possess immune-boosting properties that can help the body defend against infections, viruses, and diseases. Incorporating these herbs into your diet and wellness routine can promote overall health and resilience.

Common Herbs for Immune Support

1. Echinacea (Echinacea purpurea): Echinacea is one of the most well-known herbs for immune support. It contains compounds like echinacoside and alkylamides that stimulate the activity of immune cells, enhancing the body's defence against infections.

Uses: Echinacea is often used to prevent and treat colds, flu, and other respiratory infections. It may also help reduce the severity and duration of symptoms.

2. Elderberry (Sambucus nigra): Elderberry is rich in flavonoids, particularly anthocyanins, which have antioxidant and anti-inflammatory properties. It also contains vitamins A, C, and B6, as well as minerals like potassium and iron.

Uses: Elderberry is commonly used to support immune function and shorten the duration of colds and flu. It may help reduce congestion, coughing, and fever.

3. Astragalus (Astragalus membranaceus): Astragalus is an adaptogenic herb that supports the immune system by increasing the production of white blood cells, which play a key role in immune defence. It also has antiviral and anti-inflammatory properties.

Uses: Astragalus is often used to prevent respiratory infections, boost immunity during times of stress, and support overall vitality.

4. Garlic (Allium sativum): Garlic is a popular culinary herb with numerous therapeutic properties. Its active compound, allicin, has antibacterial, antiviral, and antifungal effects, making it beneficial for immune system support, cardiovascular health, and blood pressure regulation. Garlic may also aid in digestion and help reduce inflammation.

5. Ginger (Zingiber officinale): Ginger contains gingerol, a bioactive compound with antioxidant and anti-inflammatory properties. It also has antimicrobial properties that can help fight infections.

Uses: Ginger is commonly used to relieve nausea, digestive discomfort, and inflammation. It may also support immune function and improve circulation.

6. Turmeric (Curcuma longa): Turmeric contains curcumin, a potent antioxidant and anti-inflammatory compound. It supports immune function by modulating the activity of immune cells and reducing inflammation.

Uses: Turmeric is used to boost immunity, reduce inflammation, and support overall health. It may also help relieve joint pain, improve digestion, and protect against chronic diseases.

Herbs for Immune Support
Licorice Root (Glycyrrhiza glabra): Licorice root contains glycyrrhizin, a compound with antiviral and immune-stimulating properties. It also has anti-inflammatory and antioxidant effects.

Uses: Licorice root is used to support immune function, relieve respiratory symptoms, and soothe sore throats. It may also help improve adrenal function and support stress resilience.

Incorporating Herbs for Immune Support into Your Routine

1. Herbal Teas and Infusions: Brew immune-supportive herbs like echinacea, elderberry, and ginger into teas or infusions. Drink them regularly to boost immunity and promote overall wellness.

2. Tinctures and Extracts: Take immune-boosting herbs in tincture or extract form for concentrated doses of active compounds. Follow dosage instructions carefully and consult with a healthcare professional if needed.

3. Culinary Use: Incorporate immune-supportive herbs like garlic, ginger, and turmeric into your cooking. Add them to soups, stews, stir-fries, and other dishes for added flavour and health benefits.

4. Supplements: Consider taking herbal supplements that contain immune-supportive herbs in standardised doses. Look for high-quality products from reputable brands.

5. Topical Applications: Some herbs can be used topically to support immune function and relieve symptoms of colds and flu. For example, garlic and ginger can be infused into oils for chest rubs or added to bathwater for steam inhalation.

Safety and Considerations
1. Quality and Purity: Choose high-quality, organic herbs from reputable sources to ensure purity and potency. Avoid herbs that may be contaminated with pesticides, heavy metals, or other toxins.

2. Dosage and Administration: Follow recommended dosage guidelines for each herb and consult with a healthcare professional if you have any concerns or medical conditions.

3. Pregnancy and Medical Conditions: Some herbs may not be suitable for pregnant or breastfeeding women or individuals with certain medical conditions. Consult with a healthcare provider before using herbal remedies, especially if you are taking medications or have underlying health concerns.

4. Allergies and Sensitivities: Be aware of potential allergies or sensitivities to certain herbs. Monitor for any adverse reactions and discontinue use if you experience any symptoms.

5. Moderation: While herbs are generally safe for consumption in food amounts, excessive intake or prolonged use of certain herbs may cause gastrointestinal

Herbs for Digestive Health

Herbs have long been utilised to support and enhance digestive health due to their natural properties, including anti-inflammatory, carminative, and soothing effects on the gastrointestinal tract. Incorporating these herbs into your diet and lifestyle can promote digestion, alleviate discomfort, and support overall gastrointestinal well-being.

Common Herbs for Digestive Health

1. Peppermint (Mentha piperita): Peppermint contains menthol, which has antispasmodic properties that help relax the muscles of the digestive tract. It also soothes digestive discomfort and reduces bloating and gas.
Uses: Peppermint tea is commonly used to relieve indigestion, gas, and bloating. It may also help alleviate symptoms of irritable bowel syndrome (IBS) and promote bile flow.

2. Ginger (Zingiber officinale): Ginger contains gingerol, a bioactive compound with anti-inflammatory and carminative properties. It stimulates digestion, relieves nausea, and reduces intestinal cramping and gas.
Uses: Ginger tea or fresh ginger root can be consumed to alleviate nausea, indigestion, and motion sickness. It may also help reduce symptoms of gastrointestinal upset.

3. Chamomile (Matricaria chamomilla): Chamomile has anti-inflammatory, antispasmodic, and calming effects on the digestive system. It helps soothe the stomach, reduce acidity, and alleviate digestive discomfort.
Uses: Chamomile tea is often consumed to relieve indigestion, bloating, and abdominal cramps. It may

also promote relaxation and reduce stress-related digestive issues.

4. **Fennel (Foeniculum vulgare):** Fennel contains volatile oils like anethole, which have carminative and anti-inflammatory properties. It helps relax the gastrointestinal muscles, reduce gas, and alleviate bloating and indigestion.
Uses: Fennel tea or seeds can be consumed after meals to aid digestion and relieve gas and bloating. It may also help stimulate appetite and promote healthy bowel movements.

5. **Dandelion (Taraxacum officinale):** Dandelion root has bitter compounds that stimulate digestive juices, including bile production, which aids in the digestion of fats. It also has diuretic properties that help eliminate toxins from the body.
Uses: Dandelion root tea or supplements can be consumed to support liver and gallbladder health, improve digestion, and relieve constipation.

6. **Licorice Root (Glycyrrhiza glabra):** Licorice root contains glycyrrhizin, which has demulcent and anti-inflammatory properties that soothe and protect the mucous membranes of the digestive tract. It also supports healthy stomach acid production.
Uses: Licorice root tea or supplements are used to relieve symptoms of heartburn, acid reflux, and

gastritis. It may also help soothe throat irritation and promote ulcer healing.

7. Turmeric (Curcuma longa): Turmeric contains curcumin, a bioactive compound with anti-inflammatory and antioxidant properties. It helps reduce inflammation in the digestive tract, improve digestion, and protect against gastrointestinal diseases.

Uses: Turmeric can be added to curries, soups, and smoothies to promote digestive health. Turmeric supplements may also be taken to support overall gastrointestinal function.

Incorporating Herbs for Digestive Health into Your Routine

1. Herbal Teas: Brew digestive herbs like peppermint, ginger, chamomile, or fennel into teas and sip them before or after meals to aid digestion and relieve discomfort.

2. Herbal Supplements: Take herbal supplements containing digestive herbs in capsule or tablet form to support gastrointestinal health. Choose high-quality products from reputable brands.

3. Culinary Use: Incorporate digestive herbs like ginger, turmeric, and fennel into your cooking. Use them in soups, stews, stir-fries, or marinades to enhance flavour and promote digestion.

4. Tinctures and Extracts: Add digestive herb tinctures or extracts to water or juice and consume them before meals to stimulate digestion and reduce bloating and gas.

5. Topical Applications: Some digestive herbs can be applied topically to alleviate digestive discomfort. For example, peppermint oil can be diluted and massaged onto the abdomen to relieve gas and bloating.

Safety and Considerations
1. Quality and Purity: Choose high-quality, organic herbs from reputable sources to ensure purity and potency. Avoid herbs that may be contaminated with pesticides, heavy metals, or other toxins.

2. Dosage and Administration: Follow recommended dosage guidelines for each herb and consult with a healthcare professional if you have any concerns or medical conditions.

3. Pregnancy and Medical Conditions: Some herbs may not be suitable for pregnant or breastfeeding women or individuals with certain medical conditions. Consult with a healthcare provider before using herbal remedies, especially if you are taking medications or have underlying health concerns.

4. Allergies and Sensitivities: Be aware of potential allergies or sensitivities to certain herbs. Monitor for any adverse reactions and discontinue use if you experience any symptoms.

5. Moderation: While herbs are generally safe for consumption in food amounts, excessive intake or prolonged use of certain herbs may cause gastrointestinal discomfort. As with any dietary supplement, use herbs for digestive health in moderation and listen to your body's response.

Chapter 4: Growing Your Own Herbs

Choosing the Right Herbs for Your Garden

Choosing the right herbs for your garden involves considering factors like climate, space, purpose, and personal preferences. To select the best herbs for your garden, consider the following factors.

Factors to Consider:
1. Climate and Growing Conditions: Choose herbs that thrive in your local climate and growing conditions. Consider factors like sunlight, temperature, soil type, and water availability. Research which herbs are suitable for your hardiness zone and microclimate. Some herbs prefer full sun, while others tolerate partial shade.

2. Space and Garden Layout: Assess the available space in your garden and plan accordingly. Determine whether you'll be growing herbs in raised beds, containers, or directly in the ground. Consider the height and spread of each herb when planning their placement in the garden. Some herbs, like mint and oregano, can spread rapidly and may require containment.

3. Purpose and Use: Identify the primary purpose for growing herbs in your garden. Are you growing them for culinary use, medicinal purposes, fragrance, or ornamental value? - Select herbs that align with your intended use. For culinary gardens, prioritise herbs commonly used in cooking. For medicinal gardens, focus on herbs with therapeutic properties.

4. Companion Planting and Pest Control: Explore companion planting techniques to maximise the health and productivity of your garden. Some herbs have natural pest-repelling properties or attract beneficial insects. Consider planting herbs that deter pests or attract pollinators to create a balanced ecosystem in your garden. For example, basil repels mosquitoes, while lavender attracts bees.

5. Personal Preferences and Favourites: Choose herbs that you enjoy using and consuming. Consider your culinary preferences, favourite flavours, and aroma preferences when selecting herbs for your garden. Experiment with a variety of herbs to discover new flavours and expand your culinary repertoire. Include a mix of familiar favourites and lesser-known herbs to diversify your garden.

Popular Herbs for Home Gardens

1. Basil (Ocimum basilicum): A versatile culinary herb with a variety of cultivars offering different flavours and aromas. Basil thrives in warm, sunny conditions and is perfect for pesto, salads, and pasta dishes.

2. Rosemary (Rosmarinus officinalis): A hardy perennial herb with aromatic leaves that add flavour to roasted meats, potatoes, and bread. Rosemary prefers well-drained soil and full sun, making it ideal for Mediterranean climates.

3. Thyme (Thymus vulgaris): A low-growing herb with fragrant leaves used in soups, stews, and marinades. Thyme tolerates drought and prefers sandy, well-drained soil in full sun to partial shade.

4. Mint (Mentha spp.): Mint is a versatile and easy-to-grow herb that offers a refreshing taste and aroma. With several varieties available, such as peppermint and spearmint, mint is a popular addition to herb gardens.

5. Parsley (Petroselinum crispum): A biennial herb with flat or curly leaves used as a garnish or flavouring agent in a variety of dishes. Parsley prefers rich, well-drained soil and partial shade in hot climates.

6. Lavender (Lavandula spp.): A fragrant herb with aromatic flowers used in teas, sachets, and culinary recipes. Lavender thrives in dry, well-drained soil and full sun, making it suitable for Mediterranean gardens.

7. Chives (Allium schoenoprasum): A perennial herb with mild onion flavour used in salads, soups, and garnishes. Chives prefer fertile, well-drained soil and full sun to partial shade.

Soil, Water, and Light Requirements

Creating the right environment for your herbs to thrive involves providing the appropriate soil, water, and light conditions. Here are some general guidelines to follow.

Soil Requirements:
1. Well-Drained Soil: Herbs thrive in well-drained soil that allows excess water to drain away, preventing waterlogged conditions that can lead to root rot. Choose soil with good drainage properties, such as sandy loam or loamy soil amended with organic matter like compost or aged manure.

2. pH Level: Most herbs prefer slightly acidic to neutral soil with a pH range of 6.0 to 7.0. Conduct a soil test to determine the pH level and adjust it if necessary using lime to raise pH or sulphur to lower pH.

3. Nutrient-Rich Soil: Provide herbs with nutrient-rich soil to support healthy growth and development. Amend the soil with organic fertilisers or compost to ensure adequate levels of essential nutrients like nitrogen, phosphorus, and potassium.

4. Container Gardening: Container gardening is an excellent option for growing herbs in small spaces or for those who don't have access to a traditional garden plot.

Water Requirements
1. Consistent Moisture: Most herbs prefer consistent moisture levels in the soil, but they don't like to be waterlogged. Water herbs regularly, keeping the soil evenly moist but not soggy. - Water herbs deeply to encourage deep root growth, especially during hot weather or periods of drought.

2. Avoid Overwatering: Overwatering is a common mistake in herb gardening, as it can lead to root rot, fungal diseases, and other issues.

3. Watering Methods: Water herbs at the base of the plants to avoid wetting the foliage, which can promote fungal diseases. Use a soaker hose, drip irrigation system, or watering can with a spout for precise watering.

4. Container Watering: Check the moisture level of container-grown herbs frequently, as they may dry out more quickly than herbs planted in the ground. Water containers when the top inch of soil feels dry to the touch.

Light Requirements
1. Full Sun: Most culinary herbs thrive in full sun, receiving at least 6 to 8 hours of direct sunlight per day. Choose a sunny location for planting herbs to ensure optimal growth and productivity. Herbs grown in partial shade may have weaker flavours and slower growth rates compared to those grown in full sun.

2. Partial Shade: Some herbs, like cilantro and parsley, tolerate partial shade and can thrive in locations with dappled sunlight or morning sun followed by afternoon shade. If growing herbs indoors or in areas with limited sunlight, provide supplemental lighting using grow lights to mimic natural sunlight.

3. Indoor Gardening: When growing herbs indoors, place them near south-facing windows or under artificial grow lights to ensure they receive sufficient light for healthy growth. Rotate indoor herbs regularly to ensure even light exposure and prevent them from leaning or stretching toward the light source.

Organic Gardening Practices

Nurturing the Earth for Future Generations
Organic gardening is a philosophy that encompasses much more than the absence of synthetic chemicals. It's a commitment to creating and maintaining an ecosystem that is sustainable, resilient, and harmonious with nature. Here's an in-depth exploration.

1. Soil Stewardship: The Heart of Organic Gardening
Living Soil, Organic gardening starts with the soil. Healthy soil is teeming with life; it's a complex community of organisms, from bacteria and fungi to earthworms and insects, all playing a role in the soil's fertility and the health of plants.

2. Compost: Compost is the cornerstone of organic gardening, transforming organic waste into a rich, nutrient-dense humus that feeds the soil. It's a natural cycle of decay and renewal that enriches the soil structure, providing aeration and moisture retention.

3. Natural Fertilisers: Organic gardeners use natural fertilisers like manure, bone meal, and green manure (cover crops) to enrich the soil without the need for synthetic chemicals. These natural fertilisers release nutrients slowly, in sync with plant needs, and help to build long-term soil fertility.

Pest and Disease Management

1. A Balanced Approach: Integrated Pest Management (IPM): Organic gardening employs IPM strategies that include monitoring for pests, using natural predators and barriers, and only resorting to organic-approved pesticides as a last resort.

2. Disease Resistance: Choosing plant varieties that are resistant to diseases is a proactive way to minimise problems. These varieties have been bred to resist specific pathogens, reducing the need for interventions.

3. Diversity: A diverse garden mimics natural ecosystems, where a variety of species coexist and support each other. This diversity helps to prevent the spread of pests and diseases and creates a more resilient garden.

Water Wisdom: Conserving Life's Vital Resource
Efficient Watering: Organic gardens often utilise drip irrigation systems, which deliver water directly to the base of plants, minimising evaporation and runoff. This targeted watering approach ensures that water is used efficiently and conservatively.
Mulching: Mulch is a multi-purpose tool in the organic garden. It conserves moisture, suppresses weeds, and as it breaks down, it contributes organic matter to the soil. Organic mulches, such as straw, wood chips, or leaf litter, are preferred.

Cultivating Biodiversity: The Key to a Healthy Garden
Habitat Creation: Organic gardens often include features like hedgerows, ponds, and wildflower meadows that provide habitat for beneficial wildlife. These habitats attract and support pollinators, predators of pests, and other beneficial creatures.
Crop Rotation: Rotating crops from year to year is an age-old practice that prevents the depletion of soil nutrients and disrupts the lifecycle of pests and diseases. This practice is a fundamental aspect of maintaining a healthy and productive organic garden.

Ethical and Sustainable Practices:
Seed Sovereignty: Many organic gardeners save their own seeds or source them from ethical,

sustainable seed companies. This practice supports genetic diversity and helps preserve heirloom varieties.

Local Focus: Organic gardening often emphasises local growing, which reduces the carbon footprint associated with transporting food and supports local economies.

Community Engagement

Education: Organic gardeners often share their knowledge through workshops, community programs, and school gardens. Education is seen as a vital tool for spreading the principles of organic gardening and encouraging sustainable living.

Collaboration: Community gardens and allotments are places where organic gardeners can come together to grow food, share experiences, and build community resilience.

Challenges and Rewards:

Patience Required: Organic gardening requires patience and a willingness to learn from nature. It's a process of trial and error, observation, and adaptation.

Long-Term Benefits: While organic gardening can present challenges, the long-term benefits for the environment, human health, and the well-being of all creatures are immeasurable. Organic gardening is not just a set of practices; it's a way of life that respects the interconnectedness of all living things. It offers a path to a sustainable future, where the food we grow and eat is produced in harmony with nature.

Harvesting and Storing Herbs

Harvesting herbs is both an art and a science, requiring careful attention to timing, technique, and the specific needs of each plant.

1. Optimal Timing: The best time to harvest herbs is when their essential oils are at their highest concentration, which is typically in the morning after the dew has evaporated but before the sun is at its peak. For annual herbs, this is often just before they flower, while for perennials, it may vary depending on the plant.
Technique Matters: Use clean, sharp tools to avoid bruising the plant tissues. Snip leaves or stems above a leaf node or pair of leaves to encourage new growth. For roots, harvest in the autumn after the foliage has faded, when the plant's energy has returned to the roots.

2. Harvesting Roots: Digging up roots requires a gentle touch to avoid damaging them. Loosen the soil around the plant with a fork, then lift the roots out, shaking off excess soil, and rinse them gently.
Drying Herbs: Preserving the Essence

Drying is a critical step in preserving herbs, and there are several methods to do so, each with its own advantages.

3. Air-Drying: This traditional method involves hanging herbs in small bunches in a dry, warm place with good air circulation. An attic, shed, or even a dry room in your home can serve as a suitable drying spot. Ensure the area is out of direct sunlight to prevent the loss of potent volatile oils.

4. Screen Drying: For individual leaves or flowers, drying on screens or racks is effective. Lay the herbs out in a single layer on a mesh screen and turn them regularly to ensure even drying.

5. Dehydrator Drying: If you live in a humid climate or need to process large quantities of herbs, a dehydrator can be invaluable. Set it to the lowest setting (95°F to 115°F) to dry the herbs slowly and retain their active compounds.

6. Storing Herbs: Locking in Potency
Proper storage is essential to maintain the potency and flavour of dried herbs. Airtight Containers: Glass jars with airtight lids are ideal for storage, as they don't allow moisture or odours to penetrate. Ensure the jars are completely dry before filling them with herbs to prevent mould growth.

7. Cool, Dark, Dry: Store your containers in a cool, dark, and dry place. A cupboard away from the stove or any heat source is perfect. Light and heat can degrade the herbs quickly, so avoid sunny spots.

8. Vacuum Sealing: For long-term storage, vacuum-sealed bags can protect herbs from air and moisture. This method is particularly useful for herbs that you don't use frequently.

Freezing Herbs, Retaining Freshness : Freezing is an alternative to drying, especially for herbs that don't dry well, like basil or chives.
Ice Cube Trays: Chop the herbs and place them in ice cube trays, covering them with water or stock for use in cooking. Once frozen, transfer the cubes to a

Freezer Bags: You can also freeze whole sprigs or chopped herbs in freezer bags. Remove as much air as possible before sealing to prevent freezer burn.
Special Considerations:

Labelling: Always label your containers with the name of the herb and the date of harvest. This helps you keep track of freshness and plan your usage.

Monitoring: Check your stored herbs periodically for signs of spoilage, such as mould or a change in colour or aroma. Discard any that show signs of degradation.

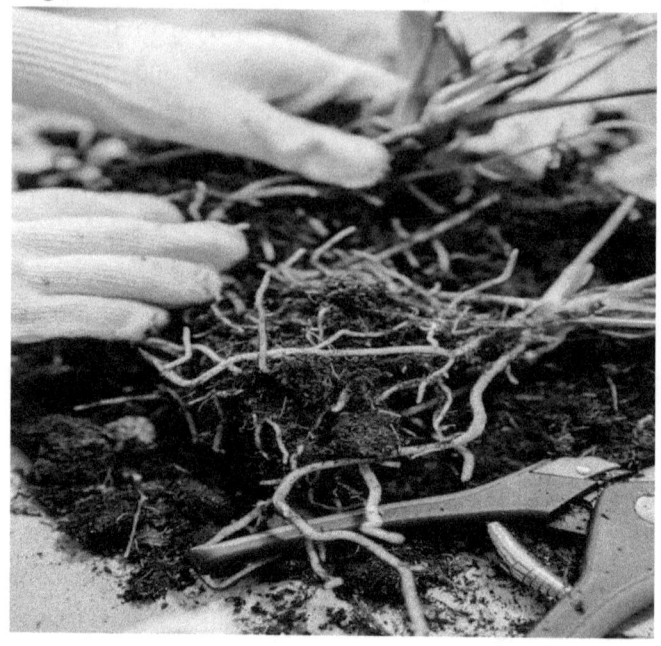

Chapter 5: Herbal Remedies for Common Ailments

Cold and Flu Relief

When it comes to finding relief from the common cold or flu, understanding the body's response to these illnesses and how various treatments can alleviate symptoms is crucial. Here's a comprehensive explanation of cold and flu relief, encompassing traditional remedies, modern medicine, and practical self-care measures.

Understanding Cold and Flu
Viral Infections: Both colds and flu are caused by viruses, with the common cold often attributed to rhinoviruses, while the flu is caused by influenza viruses.
Symptoms: While both can produce similar symptoms, flu symptoms are generally more severe and can include fever, body aches, extreme tiredness, and dry cough. Colds tend to be milder and are more likely to cause a runny or stuffy nose.

The Role of the Immune System: The immune system is the body's primary defence against viral infections. It uses a complex network of cells and proteins to identify and neutralise foreign invaders.

Inflammation: Part of the immune response includes inflammation, which, while a natural part of healing, can also cause discomfort and symptoms like swelling, redness, and pain.

Herbal Remedies for Symptom Relief: Studies suggest that echinacea can reduce the chances of developing a cold and may shorten its duration. It's thought to work by stimulating the immune system.
Elderberry: Elderberry is rich in vitamins and antioxidants. It's been shown to reduce the severity and length of flu symptoms when taken within 48 hours of the first symptoms.
Ginger: Ginger has anti-inflammatory properties that can help soothe a sore throat, reduce nausea, and lower fever. Ginger tea is a comforting way to take this remedy.
Supportive Nutrients: Vitamin C: While vitamin C hasn't been shown to prevent colds, it may reduce the severity and duration of symptoms.
Zinc: Zinc can help reduce the duration of cold symptoms if taken soon after they appear. Zinc lozenges or syrups are commonly used for this purpose.
Adequate Sleep: Getting enough sleep is vital for the immune system to fight off the virus effectively.
Reduced Activity: Resting allows the body to direct more energy toward the immune response rather than

toward other physically demanding activities. Over-the-Counter.
Medications: Pain Relievers: Acetaminophen or ibuprofen can help alleviate fever, sore throat, and headaches.
Cough Suppressants: Medications like dextromethorphan can reduce the urge to cough.
Home Care Practices: Steam Inhalation: Breathing in steam can moisten the upper airways and provide relief from congestion.
Saltwater Gargle: Gargling with salt water can soothe a sore throat and reduce mucus.
Humidifiers: Using a humidifier adds moisture to the air, which can ease congestion and coughing.

Prevention and Precautions: Hand Hygiene, Regular hand washing is one of the most effective ways to prevent the spread of cold and flu viruses. **Flu Vaccine**: An annual flu vaccine is the best way to reduce the chances of getting the flu and spreading it to others. When to Seek Medical **Attention, Severe Symptoms**: High or prolonged fever, difficulty breathing, chest pain, or severe weakness are signs that medical attention is needed. **At-Risk Groups:** Young children, the elderly, pregnant women, and those with chronic health conditions should consult a healthcare provider early in the course of the illness.

Headache and Migraine Remedies

Headaches and migraines are common neurological conditions that can range from mild discomfort to severe pain, significantly impacting daily life. Understanding the nuances of these conditions and the variety of available remedies is crucial for effective management and relief. Here's an extensive exploration of the topic.

Headaches: Types and Triggers Tension Headaches. The most common type, characterised by a dull, aching sensation all over the head, often accompanied by tenderness in the shoulders, neck, or scalp.

Cluster Headaches: Intense, piercing pain on one side of the head; they occur in groups or "clusters" over a period. Sinus.
Headaches: Caused by inflammation of the sinuses, these headaches are felt as a deep and constant pain in the cheekbones, forehead, or bridge of the nose.
Migraines: A more severe form of headache, migraines are often accompanied by other symptoms such as nausea, vomiting, and extreme sensitivity to light and sound.
Migraine Specifics, Aura: Some people experience 'aura' before a migraine, which can include visual

disturbances, tingling in the arms or legs, or difficulty speaking.

Phases: Migraines typically progress through four stages: prodrome, aura, attack, and postdrome, each with distinct symptoms.

Common Triggers

Food and Drinks: Certain foods and beverages, like aged cheeses, processed foods, alcohol, and caffeine, can trigger headaches and migraines. **Stress:** High levels of stress or even the period of relaxation after stress (known as the "let-down effect") can precipitate headaches.

Sensory Stimuli: Bright lights, loud sounds, and strong smells can trigger migraines in sensitive individuals.

Changes in Sleep: Both lack of sleep and oversleeping can serve as triggers.

Environmental Changes: Weather changes, barometric pressure variations, and altitude changes are potential triggers.

Herbal and Natural Remedies: Feverfew (Tanacetum parthenium) A traditional remedy for migraines, feverfew is thought to reduce inflammation and prevent blood vessel constriction.

Butterbur (Petasites hybridus): Studies suggest butterbur can reduce the frequency of migraine attacks, possibly due to its anti-inflammatory effects.

Peppermint Oil: Applied topically, peppermint oil can create a cooling sensation that may relieve tension headaches.

Ginger: Known for its anti-inflammatory properties, ginger can alleviate nausea and may reduce the severity of migraine headaches.

Nutritional Interventions: Magnesium: Deficiency in magnesium has been linked to headaches and migraines. Supplements or magnesium-rich foods like almonds, spinach, and avocados can help.

Riboflavin (Vitamin B2): High doses of riboflavin have been shown to reduce migraine frequency in some people.

Coenzyme Q10: This enzyme plays a role in energy production and may be beneficial in reducing migraine occurrence. Lifestyle Modifications: Stress **Management:** Techniques such as meditation, progressive muscle relaxation, and biofeedback can help manage stress and reduce headache frequency.

Regular Exercise: Physical activity can reduce the frequency and intensity of migraines by releasing endorphins, the body's natural painkillers. Adequate **Hydration:** Dehydration can trigger headaches, so it's important to drink plenty of fluids throughout the day. Medical Treatments: Over-the-Counter Pain **Relievers:** NSAIDs or acetaminophen can provide relief for mild headaches.

Triptans: Prescription medications specifically for migraines, triptans work by constricting blood

vessels and blocking pain pathways in the brain.
Preventive Medications: For chronic migraine sufferers, medications such as beta-blockers, antidepressants, or anticonvulsants may be prescribed to reduce the frequency and severity of migraines.
Complementary Therapies: Acupuncture: This traditional Chinese medicine technique has been shown to be effective in reducing headache frequency and severity.
Massage Therapy: Regular massages can help reduce stress and tension, which may, in turn, decrease the occurrence of headaches.

Environmental Adjustments
Ergonomic Workspaces: Proper posture and ergonomic office setups can prevent headaches caused by muscle strain.
Lighting: For those sensitive to light, using anti-glare screens, sunglasses, and dimming lights can help. When to Seek Professional Help: New or **Worsening Symptoms:** If headaches change in pattern or intensity, it's important to consult a healthcare provider. Frequent or Severe **Headaches:** Persistent or severe headaches warrant medical evaluation to rule out underlying conditions.

Digestive Disorders and Solutions

Digestive disorders encompass a broad spectrum of conditions that can affect any part of the gastrointestinal (GI) tract. Understanding these conditions and their respective solutions is essential for managing symptoms and maintaining digestive health. Here's an extensive exploration of common digestive disorders and their potential solutions.

Irritable Bowel Syndrome (IBS): IBS is characterised by a combination of symptoms such as abdominal pain, bloating, and changes in bowel habits (constipation, diarrhoea, or both). **Management Strategies:** Dietary adjustments (low FODMAP diet), probiotics, fibre supplements, antispasmodic medications, and psychological therapies like cognitive-behavioural therapy (CBT) or hypnotherapy.

Gastroesophageal Reflux Disease (GERD): GERD occurs when stomach acid frequently flows back into the tube connecting the mouth and stomach (oesophagus). This backwash (acid reflux) can irritate the lining of the oesophagus.
Management Strategies: Lifestyle modifications (weight loss, elevating the head of the bed, avoiding late meals), dietary changes (limiting acidic and

spicy foods), over-the-counter antacids, H2 receptor blockers, proton pump inhibitors (PPIs), and in severe cases, surgical interventions.

Inflammatory Bowel Disease (IBD): IBD primarily includes Crohn's disease and ulcerative colitis, which are characterised by chronic inflammation of the GI tract.
Management Strategies: Anti-inflammatory drugs (aminosalicylates, corticosteroids), immune system suppressors, biologics, antibiotics, dietary management, and surgery to remove damaged sections of the GI tract or to treat complications.

Celiac Disease: An immune reaction to eating gluten, a protein found in wheat, barley, and rye.
Management Strategies: A strict gluten-free diet is the primary treatment. Nutritional support may be necessary to address any deficiencies.

Peptic Ulcers: Proton pump inhibitors, H2 receptor blockers, antibiotics to treat Helicobacter pylori infection, and protective medications to shield the stomach's lining.
Gallstones: Hardened deposits of digestive fluid that can form in the gallbladder.
Management Strategies: Medications to dissolve gallstones, surgical removal of the gallbladder

(cholecystectomy), and lifestyle changes to reduce cholesterol intake.

Pancreatitis: Inflammation of the pancreas, which can occur as acute pancreatitis or chronic pancreatitis.
Management Strategies: Hospitalisation for acute cases to rest the pancreas, pain management, IV fluids, and nutritional support. Chronic pancreatitis may require enzyme supplements and dietary changes.

Functional Dyspepsia: Persistent or recurring indigestion with no clear cause.
Management Strategies: Dietary modifications, medications to reduce stomach acid, prokinetics, and psychological therapies. General Digestive Health

Dietary Fibre: A high-fibre diet helps to keep food moving through the digestive tract, reducing the risk of constipation and associated disorders.
Regular Exercise: Physical activity helps maintain regular bowel movements.
Mindful Eating: Eating slowly and chewing thoroughly aids digestion and can prevent overeating, which may trigger digestive discomfort.
Avoiding Triggers: Identifying and avoiding specific foods or beverages that trigger symptoms can help manage many digestive disorders.

Stress Reduction: Chronic stress can negatively impact digestive health, so incorporating stress-reduction techniques can be beneficial.

When to Seek Medical Attention: Persistent Symptoms: If digestive symptoms are persistent, worsening, or affecting quality of life, it's important to seek medical evaluation.

Red Flags: Symptoms such as unexplained weight loss, blood in stool, difficulty swallowing, or persistent vomiting require immediate medical attention. It's important to note that while lifestyle changes and dietary adjustments can significantly improve digestive health, they should be tailored to individual needs and conditions. Working with healthcare professionals, including gastroenterologists and dietitians, can ensure that management strategies are effective and appropriate for the specific digestive disorder.

Skin Conditions and Treatments

Skin conditions like eczema, psoriasis, acne, and rosacea cause discomfort. Herbal remedies such as calendula, chamomile, aloe vera, and tea tree oil can soothe symptoms. Consult a healthcare professional. Here's a detailed look at some common skin conditions and their treatments.

Acne: Causes: Acne is caused by clogged hair follicles due to oil and dead skin cells. It's common in teenagers but can occur at any age. Symptoms: It presents as redness, blackheads, whiteheads, pimples, or painful cysts and nodules.

Treatments: Over-the-counter topical treatments, prescription medications, hormonal therapy, and lifestyle changes like diet and stress management.

Eczema (Atopic Dermatitis): The exact cause is unknown, but it's believed to be linked to an overactive immune system response to irritants.
Symptoms: Itchy inflammation, red or brownish-grey patches, small raised bumps, and cracked or scaly skin.
Treatments: Moisturizing creams, topical corticosteroids, antihistamines, and avoiding triggers1.
Psoriasis: An autoimmune condition that speeds up the growth cycle of skin cells.
Symptoms: Red patches covered with thick, silvery scales, dry or cracked skin that may bleed, itching or soreness.
Treatments: Topical treatments, phototherapy, systemic medications, and biologics1.

Rosacea: The cause of rosacea is not fully understood but may be related to hereditary and environmental factors.

Symptoms: Facial redness, swollen red bumps, visible blood vessels, and eye problems.
Treatments: Topical medications, oral antibiotics, laser therapy, and identifying and avoiding triggers.

Melanoma (Skin Cancer): Caused by mutations in the DNA of skin cells, often due to UV radiation from sunlight or tanning beds.
Symptoms: New or changing moles, pigmented lesions, and unusual growths on the skin.
Treatments: Surgical removal, chemotherapy, radiation therapy, targeted therapy, and immunotherapy.

Contact Dermatitis: An allergic reaction to something that touches the skin, such as certain soaps, cosmetics, fragrances, jewellery, or plants.
Symptoms: Red rash, itching, dry or cracked skin, bumps and blisters, and swelling. Treatments: Avoiding the allergen, corticosteroid creams, oral medications, and cool compresses.

Vitiligo: An autoimmune disorder where the immune system attacks and destroys the melanocytes in the skin.
Symptoms: Loss of skin colour in patches, premature whitening of hair, and loss of colour in the tissues inside the mouth.

Treatments: Phototherapy, topical corticosteroids, skin camouflage, and in some cases, surgery1.

Hives (Urticaria): Often due to an allergic reaction to medication, food, or other irritants.
Symptoms: Red, itchy welts on the skin, which may vary in size and shape.
Treatments: Antihistamines, avoiding known triggers, and corticosteroids for severe cases1.

Shingles (Herpes Zoster): Caused by the reactivation of the varicella-zoster virus, which causes chickenpox.
Symptoms: Painful rash, blisters, itching, fever, and headache.
Treatments: Antiviral medications, pain relief, and the shingles vaccine to prevent future occurrences1.

Alopecia Areata: An autoimmune disorder that attacks hair follicles.
Symptoms: Sudden hair loss that starts with one or more circular bald patches.
Treatments: Corticosteroids, minoxidil, and other medications that promote hair growth or affect the immune system1. For all skin conditions, it's important to consult with a dermatologist for an accurate diagnosis and appropriate treatment plan. Treatments can vary widely depending on the specific condition and individual factors.

Additionally, some skin conditions may be indicative of underlying health issues, so seeking professional medical advice is crucial. The information provided here is based on general knowledge about skin conditions and should not replace professional medical advice. If you're experiencing symptoms of a skin condition, please consult with a healthcare provider for an accurate diagnosis and appropriate treatment.

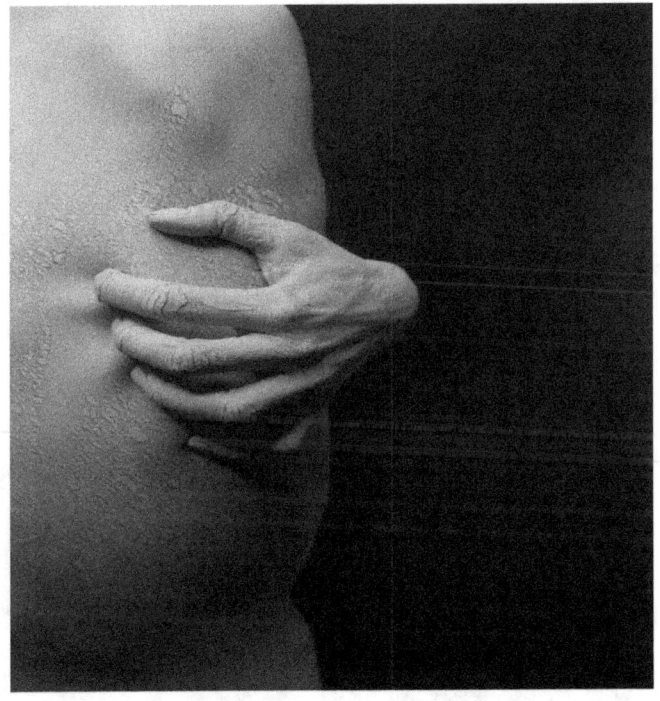

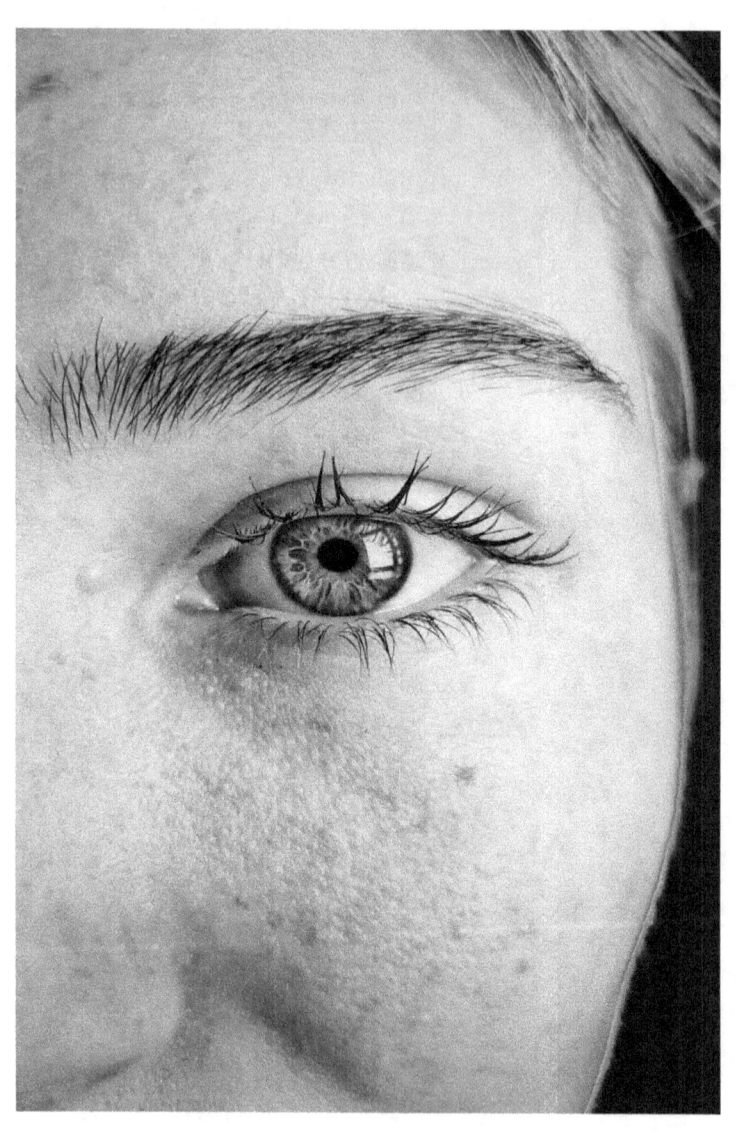

Chapter 6: Herbal Remedies for Mental Health

Herbs for Stress Relief

Herbs for Stress Relief In the fast-paced world we live in, stress has become a common companion in our daily lives. However, nature offers a bounty of herbal allies that can help soothe the mind and bring balance to our stress responses. Below are some of the most effective herbs known for their stress-relieving properties.

Ashwagandha (Withania somnifera): Often referred to as Indian ginseng, ashwagandha is a revered adaptogen in Ayurvedic medicine. It helps the body manage stress by modulating the release of stress hormones. It's known for its ability to enhance stamina and reduce anxiety.

Lavender (Lavandula angustifolia): The scent of lavender alone can act as a calming agent. It's widely used in aromatherapy for its relaxing effects and is also taken orally to help with anxiety, insomnia, and restlessness.

Chamomile (Matricaria chamomilla): is a versatile medicinal plant that belongs to the Asteraceae family. It is native to Europe and Western

Asia and has been used for centuries for its therapeutic properties.

Holy Basil (Ocimum sanctum): Also known as Tulsi, holy basil is another adaptogen that helps the body adapt to stress and promotes mental balance. It is considered a sacred plant in India and is used to support a healthy response to stress, natural detoxification, and restore balance and harmony.

Lemon Balm (Melissa officinalis): This citrus-scented herb is used in traditional medicine to improve mood and cognitive function. Lemon balm can ease stress and help with sleep due to its mild sedative effect.

Rhodiola (Rhodiola rosea): Rhodiola is notable for its ability to decrease fatigue and improve resilience to stress. This herb works by influencing key brain chemicals, such as serotonin and dopamine, which play a role in mood regulation and cognitive function. Incorporating these herbs into wellness routines can be a cornerstone for a health-focused business. Products such as teas, supplements, and essential oils derived from these herbs are in high demand as people increasingly seek natural ways to manage stress.

Enhancing Mood with Herbs

Enhancing Mood with Herbs The quest for happiness is as old as humanity itself, and in our modern era, the use of herbs to uplift the spirit is gaining popularity. Herbs can be a natural way to enhance mood, combat depression, and increase feelings of well-being. Here are some herbs known for their mood-boosting properties.

St. John's Wort (Hypericum perforatum): This herb has been used for centuries to treat mental health conditions. It's most commonly used for depression and conditions that sometimes go along with depression such as anxiety, tiredness, loss of appetite and trouble sleeping.

Saffron (Crocus sativus): Known as the 'sunshine spice', saffron is not only prized for its flavour but also for its potential antidepressant properties. Studies suggest that saffron may improve mood, reduce symptoms of depression, and increase levels of serotonin in the brain. Ginkgo Biloba Ginkgo has a long history of being used in traditional medicine to treat blood disorders and improve memory. It's also known for its ability to enhance brain function and mood.

Passionflower (Passiflora incarnata): Traditionally used to treat anxiety and insomnia, passionflower can have a calming effect, making it useful for alleviating stress and improving mood. By offering high-quality herbal products, such as capsules, extracts, or blends, and combining them with compelling educational content.

Herbal Solutions for Anxiety

Herbal Solutions for Anxiety Anxiety is a common condition that affects millions worldwide, prompting many to seek natural remedies for relief. The herbal kingdom offers a variety of plants that can help ease the mind and reduce the symptoms of anxiety. Here's a detailed exploration of some key herbs.

Valerian Root (Valeriana officinalis): Valerian root is widely recognized for its sedative qualities and its ability to relieve anxiety and improve sleep quality. Its active compounds interact with gamma-aminobutyric acid (GABA), a chemical messenger that helps regulate nerve impulses in your brain and nervous system.

Kava Kava (Piper methysticum): Kava kava is known for its calming effects, offering relief from anxiety and stress. It works by affecting the brain's neurotransmitters that modulate mood and has been used in traditional Pacific Island medicine for centuries.

CBD (Cannabidiol): Derived from the hemp plant, CBD has gained immense popularity for its anxiolytic properties without the psychoactive effects of THC. It interacts with the body's endocannabinoid system to help reduce anxiety and promote relaxation. Theanine Found in green tea leaves, theanine is an amino acid that promotes relaxation and reduces stress without causing drowsiness. It's thought to work by increasing levels of GABA, serotonin, and dopamine.

Herbal Support for Sleep Disorders

Herbal Support for Sleep Disorders A restful night's sleep is the cornerstone of good health, yet many find it elusive. The herbal realm offers a treasure trove of remedies that can support sleep without the side effects often associated with pharmaceutical sleep aids. Here's a how herbs can be used to combat sleep disorders.

Valerian (Valeriana officinalis): Valerian is perhaps the most well-known herb for sleep. It acts as a sedative on the brain and nervous system, making it a popular choice for those with insomnia.

Lavender (Lavandula angustifolia): Lavender's calming aroma is not just for fragrances; it can also be used in a pillow spray or essential oil diffuser to create a soothing sleep environment.

Passionflower (Passiflora incarnata): Traditionally used for its calming effects, passionflower can be taken as a tea or extract to help reduce nighttime awakenings and improve sleep quality.

Lemon Balm (Melissa officinalis) Lemon balm, often combined with other calming herbs, can help reduce stress and anxiety, leading to better sleep. The sleep wellness industry is thriving, and herbal sleep aids represent a growing niche.

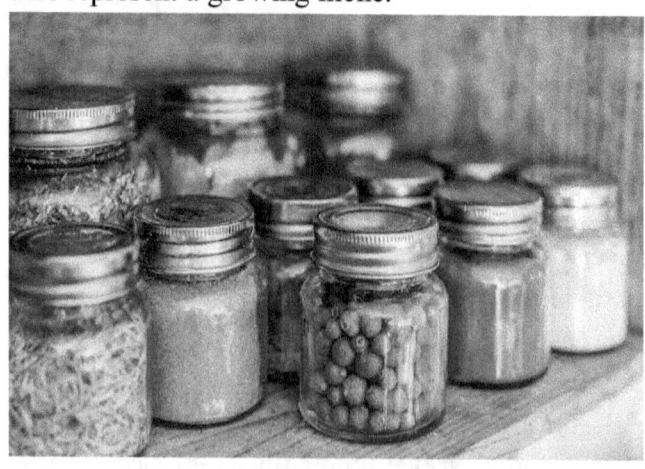

Chapter 7: Herbal Remedies for Women's Health

Hormonal Balance

Hormonal Balance for Sleep Sleep is not just a matter of closing one's eyes; it's a complex process regulated by an intricate dance of hormones. Achieving hormonal balance is key to unlocking restorative sleep. Here's how hormones affect sleep.

Melatonin: The Sleep Regulator Melatonin is the hormone most closely associated with sleep. Produced by the pineal gland, it signals the body to prepare for sleep as the light dims. Supplements that support natural melatonin production can be a cornerstone of a sleep-focused product line.

Cortisol: The Stress Hormone Cortisol should naturally decline at night, allowing for restful sleep. However, stress can disrupt this cycle. Products that help manage stress, such as adaptogenic herb supplements, can be marketed to those looking to balance their cortisol levels for better sleep.

Oestrogen and Progesterone: The Female Sleep Architects These hormones fluctuate throughout a woman's life and can significantly impact sleep quality. Offering herbal supplements that support the balance of oestrogen and progesterone can cater to a female audience seeking sleep solutions.

Testosterone: The Energy Hormone In men, low levels of testosterone can lead to sleep disturbances. Products aimed at supporting healthy testosterone levels can be targeted towards men who are experiencing sleep issues. By creating a line of supplements, teas, or even educational courses on hormonal balance for sleep, you can tap into the health and wellness industry's lucrative sleep aid segment.

Herbal Support for Menstruation and Menopause

Herbal Support for Menstruation and Menopause The transition through menstruation and menopause is a natural part of a woman's life cycle. Herbs can play a supportive role in managing symptoms and promoting hormonal balance during these times. Here's a how herbs can be used to support menstruation and menopause.

For Menstruation: Chaste Tree Berry (Vitex agnus-castus) Chaste tree berry is known for its ability to regulate menstrual cycles and ease premenstrual syndrome (PMS) symptoms by normalising the balance of female hormones. Red Raspberry Leaf (Rubus idaeus) Rich in vitamins and minerals, red raspberry leaf is traditionally used to strengthen the uterine muscles, which can help reduce menstrual cramps. Ginger (Zingiber officinale) Ginger has anti-inflammatory properties that can alleviate menstrual pain. It's also beneficial for relieving nausea, a common symptom of PMS.

For Menopause: Black Cohosh (Actaea racemosa) Black cohosh is widely used for menopause symptoms such as hot flashes, night sweats, and mood swings. It's believed to work by affecting serotonin receptors and mimicking the effects of oestrogen. Dong Quai (Angelica sinensis) Often called 'female ginseng', dong quai is used in traditional Chinese medicine to manage menopausal symptoms and improve overall vitality. Soy Isoflavones Soy contains isoflavones, which are plant-based compounds with oestrogen-like effects. They can help balance hormone levels and ease menopausal symptoms. Creating a line of herbal products tailored to women's health, especially for menstruation and menopause. These products can range from teas and capsules to topical creams and oils.

Fertility and Pregnancy

Fertility: refers to the ability to conceive or produce offspring. It encompasses various factors that influence the reproductive process, such as the quality of eggs and sperm, hormonal balance, and overall health. Fertility is essential for individuals who wish to start or expand their families.

Pregnancy: is the state in which a female carries a developing embryo or foetus in her uterus. This process begins with the fertilisation of an egg by a sperm and typically lasts around 40 weeks, during which the foetus grows and develops. Pregnancy is a complex and beautiful process that involves physiological changes and adaptations to support the growing foetus.

1. Fertility Support Products: Develop and market dietary supplements, herbal formulations, or nutrient-rich blends that support fertility and reproductive health. These products can contain ingredients such as omega-3 fatty acids, CoQ10, and antioxidants that promote optimal reproductive function. To create effective products, consider collaborating with healthcare professionals specialising in fertility, ensuring your offerings are evidence-based and cater to specific fertility concerns. This can include targeted supplements for women with irregular menstrual cycles or men with low sperm count.

2. Prenatal and Postnatal Care: Offer products or services tailored to the needs of pregnant women and new mothers. Partner with experienced yoga instructors to provide prenatal yoga classes that help improve flexibility, reduce stress, and strengthen muscles for childbirth. Additionally, provide pregnancy massage services to alleviate discomfort associated with pregnancy, such as back pain, swelling, and fatigue. Offer postpartum recovery programs focusing on physical healing, mental well-being, and baby care to support new mothers during this transformative period.

3. Education and Resources: Provide comprehensive educational resources on fertility, conception, pregnancy, and postpartum care. This can include creating a blog with informative articles, hosting webinars featuring expert speakers, or offering online courses to deepen understanding of these topics. Build a supportive online community where individuals can share experiences, seek advice, and connect with others going through similar challenges. This fosters a sense of belonging and encourages ongoing engagement with your brand.

4. Fertility and Pregnancy Coaching: Offer personalised coaching services focusing on nutrition, exercise, stress management, and environmental factors that impact fertility and pregnancy. Provide virtual consultations, allowing clients to access expert guidance from the comfort of their homes. Group workshops can provide additional peer support and create opportunities for participants to learn from each other's experiences. Develop personalised plans catering to individual needs, ensuring clients receive tailored advice to optimise their chances of conceiving or managing pregnancy.

5. Fertility Tracking Apps: Develop innovative apps that assist users in tracking their menstrual cycles, ovulation, and fertility windows to optimise conception. Integrate features like basal body temperature tracking and cervical mucus monitoring to help users identify their most fertile periods. Incorporate period prediction tools that allow women to plan for their next cycle and better understand their body's natural rhythms. Ensure the app is user-friendly, accessible, and secure to encourage widespread adoption.

Postpartum and Lactation Support

Postpartum and Lactation Support The postpartum period is a time of significant adjustment and recovery for new mothers. Herbal remedies can offer gentle support during this phase, particularly in aiding recovery and supporting lactation. Here's a how herbs can be beneficial for postpartum recovery and lactation.

For Postpartum Recovery: Nettle (Urtica dioica) Nettle is rich in vitamins and minerals, especially iron, which can be beneficial for postpartum women recovering from childbirth and looking to replenish lost nutrients. Motherwort (Leonurus cardiaca) Motherwort is traditionally used to help with the emotional and hormonal changes during the postpartum period. It's known for its calming properties and support of the heart and nerves.

For Lactation Support: Fenugreek (Trigonella foenum-graecum) Fenugreek is one of the most popular herbs for increasing milk supply. It's often found in lactation teas and supplements. Blessed Thistle (Cnicus benedictus) Blessed thistle is commonly used in combination with fenugreek to enhance breast milk production. Fennel (Foeniculum vulgare) Fennel is another herb that can help increase milk supply and is also believed to relieve colic in breastfed babies. The market for postpartum and lactation products is substantial, as new mothers seek natural ways to support their recovery and breastfeeding journey. By offering a range of herbal products, such as teas, capsules, or lactation cookies, you can provide valuable solutions to this demographic.

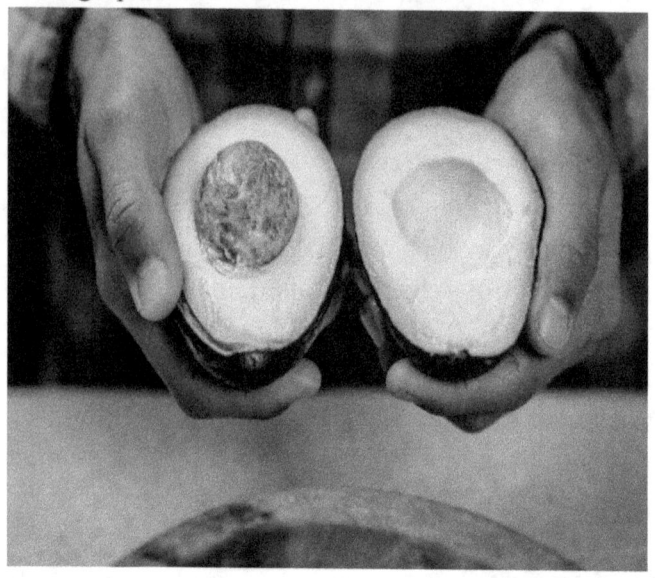

Chapter 8: Herbal Remedies for Men's Health

Prostate Health

The prostate is a small gland in men that plays a crucial role in the reproductive system. Maintaining its health is vital for urinary function and sexual health. As men age, the prostate can enlarge, leading to conditions such as Benign Prostatic Hyperplasia (BPH), which affects the quality of life.

Natural Medicine and Herbal Remedies Natural medicine offers a holistic approach to health, emphasising the body's ability to heal itself with the support of natural substances. In the context of prostate health, herbal remedies can be used to manage symptoms and support the prostate's normal function. For example, saw palmetto is a well-known herb that has been traditionally used to support prostate health and may help manage symptoms of BPH. Lifestyle and Dietary Tips In addition to herbal remedies, lifestyle changes can significantly impact prostate health. Regular exercise, a balanced diet rich in fruits and vegetables, and adequate water intake are essential for overall well-being and prostate health. Foods rich in antioxidants and omega-3 fatty acids are particularly beneficial.

Enhancing Libido and Stamina

A Key to Men's Well-being The prostate gland, a pivotal part of the male reproductive system, is often likened to a walnut in size and shape. Prostate health is a matter of considerable importance, particularly as men enter middle age and beyond, when the risk of prostate-related issues increases.

Common Prostate Conditions
Benign Prostatic Hyperplasia (BPH): This non-cancerous enlargement of the prostate can impede the flow of urine, leading to symptoms such as frequent urination, difficulty starting and stopping urine flow, and incomplete bladder emptying.

Prostatitis: An inflammation of the prostate, often caused by bacterial infection, can result in pain, difficulty urinating, and sexual dysfunction. Prostate

Cancer: The most serious condition affecting the prostate, it requires early detection and treatment. Herbal Remedies and Their Role Natural medicine advocates for the use of herbs to support prostate health. Some herbs that have been traditionally used and studied for their potential benefits include.

Saw Palmetto: Often used for BPH, it may help reduce urinary symptoms and is considered a first-line herbal treatment.

Pygeum: Derived from the African plum tree, it's used for reducing inflammation and improving urinary symptoms associated with an enlarged prostate.

Stinging Nettle: Works synergistically with other herbs to alleviate symptoms of BPH and may have anti-inflammatory properties. Integrating Herbal Remedies into Daily Life, this book guide readers on how to incorporate these herbs into their daily routine, whether through teas, supplements, or tinctures. It's essential to emphasise the importance of quality sourcing and the potential interactions with medications. The Holistic Approach A holistic view on health doesn't stop at herbal remedies. Diet, exercise, and stress management play crucial roles in maintaining prostate health. Foods rich in zinc, such as pumpkin seeds and oysters, and those with anti-inflammatory properties, like tomatoes and berries, are particularly beneficial. Navigating the Path to Wellness, readers should consult with healthcare professionals before starting any new herbal regimen, especially if they have pre-existing conditions or are taking other medications.

Herbs for Heart Health

Nature's Support for a Strong Heart The heart, our life-sustaining pump, requires proper care and nutrition to function optimally. In the realm of natural medicine, various herbs have been recognized for their heart-healthy properties. These herbs can complement a heart-conscious lifestyle that includes a balanced diet and regular exercise.

Key Herbs for Cardiovascular Support
Turmeric: Known for its vibrant colour and presence in curries, turmeric contains curcumin, a compound with anti-inflammatory and antioxidant properties. It's been found to have cardiovascular protective effects, which may help reduce the risk of heart disease.

Ginger: This versatile spice is not only a flavour enhancer but also has cholesterol-lowering properties. Ginger can improve liver function and reduce blood pressure, both of which are beneficial for heart health.

Cinnamon: With its sweet and warming flavour, cinnamon is more than just a baking ingredient. It has antioxidant, anti-inflammatory, and antidiabetic properties, which can contribute to a healthy heart by lowering cholesterol and regulating blood sugar levels.

Garlic: A staple in many cuisines, garlic has been shown to have a positive impact on various aspects of cardiovascular health, including hypertension and dyslipidemia.

Managing Stress and Vitality

Harnessing Herbal Wisdom for Stress Management and Vitality In today's fast-paced world, stress is a common ailment that can sap our energy and vitality. However, nature offers a bounty of herbs that can help us manage stress and boost our overall vitality.

Key Herbs for Stress Relief and Vitality
Ashwagandha: Known as a powerful adaptogen, ashwagandha helps the body resist and recover from stress. It's believed to improve energy levels and reduce cortisol, the stress hormone.

Rhodiola Rosea: Another adaptogen, Rhodiola Rosea, is renowned for enhancing mental performance, especially during periods of stress. It also helps fight fatigue and improve mood.

Holy Basil (Tulsi): This sacred herb is revered in Ayurvedic medicine for its ability to foster clear thoughts and relaxation. It's also said to have anti-anxiety and antidepressant properties.

Lemon Balm: With its calming scent, lemon balm can help ease stress and anxiety. It's often used to promote sleep and improve symptoms of restlessness. Integrating Herbs into Daily Routines this book provides readers with practical ways to include these herbs in their daily lives, such as through teas, tinctures, or supplements. It's important to highlight the need for consistency to see the benefits. A Holistic Approach to Stress Management Beyond herbs, a holistic approach to managing stress includes regular exercise, meditation, and a balanced diet. Techniques like deep breathing, yoga, and mindfulness can also play a significant role in reducing stress levels and enhancing vitality. Safety and Precautions While these herbs are generally safe, it's crucial to advise readers to consult with healthcare professionals before starting any new herbal regimen, especially if they are on medication or have existing health conditions.

Chapter 9: Herbal Remedies for Children

Safe Herbs for Children

When considering herbal remedies for children, it's essential to approach with a blend of caution, knowledge, and respect for the delicate nature of a child's body. Here's an extensive exploration of safe herbs for children and how they can be integrated into their healthcare. The Delicate Nature of Pediatric Herbalism Pediatric herbalism requires an understanding of how children's metabolic rates, immune systems, and organ functions differ from adults. This understanding is crucial when selecting herbs and determining dosages.

A Spectrum of Safe Herbs for Children
Chamomile (Matricaria recutita): A gentle herb that can alleviate digestive discomfort, reduce anxiety, and promote sleep. It's particularly useful for teething infants and colicky babies.

Lemon Balm (Melissa officinalis): With its mild sedative properties, lemon balm can help children suffering from nervousness or insomnia. It's also beneficial for soothing stomach issues.

Fennel (Foeniculum vulgare): Known for its antispasmodic effects, fennel can relieve gas and support digestion in children.

Ginger (Zingiber officinale): A well-known remedy for nausea and vomiting; ginger can be given in small doses to alleviate motion sickness or digestive upset.

Echinacea (Echinacea spp.): Often used to boost the immune system; Echinacea can be helpful in preventing and shortening the duration of colds.

Calendula (Calendula officinalis): Applied topically, calendula is excellent for healing skin irritations, minor wounds, and diaper rash. Dosage Considerations, Children's dosages should be carefully calculated based on weight rather than age. A common method is to use Clark's rule or Young's rule to determine the child's dose from the adult dosage.

Preparation Methods Herbal remedies for children often come in the form of teas, syrups, or glycerites. These preparations allow for easier dosing adjustments and are generally more palatable for young taste buds.

Safety Protocols, Safety is the top priority when using herbs with children. This includes:

Choosing herbs with a high safety profile.

Consulting with healthcare professionals before starting any herbal treatment.
Being aware of potential allergic reactions or side effects.
Avoiding herbs that are contraindicated in children.
Educational Resources for Parents this book provide parents with resources such as dosing charts, preparation instructions, and signs to watch for that indicate an adverse reaction. Include interviews with paediatric herbalists and healthcare professionals to add credibility.

Remedies for Common Childhood Illnesses

Herbal Allies for Childhood Ailments Children are prone to a variety of common illnesses as their immune systems develop. Herbal remedies can be gentle yet effective options for parents looking to alleviate their children's symptoms naturally.

Colds and Respiratory Infections Elderberry (Sambucus nigra): Rich in antioxidants, elderberry syrup is popular for its immune-boosting properties and can help reduce the duration and severity of colds.

Thyme (Thymus vulgaris): Thyme has antiseptic properties and can be used in a tea or as a chest rub (in an oil base) to help ease coughs and respiratory infections.

Digestive Issues Peppermint (Mentha piperita): Peppermint tea can relieve indigestion, gas, and stomach pain. It's also cooling and refreshing, which can be soothing during fevers.

Slippery Elm (Ulmus rubra): The mucilage from slippery elm can coat the digestive tract, providing relief from acid reflux and gastrointestinal irritation.

Skin Conditions Calendula (Calendula officinalis): As mentioned earlier, calendula is excellent for skin issues. It can be used in creams or lotions to soothe eczema, diaper rash, and minor cuts.

Plantain (Plantago major): Plantain leaves can be made into a poultice for insect bites, stings, and scrapes due to their anti-inflammatory and wound-healing properties.

Sleep Disturbances Lavender (Lavandula angustifolia): The calming scent of lavender can aid in relaxation and sleep. It can be used in a diffuser or as a pillow spray for children having trouble sleeping.

Teething and Pain Relief Cloves (Syzygium aromaticum): Clove oil, diluted in a carrier oil, can be applied to the gums to relieve teething pain due to its natural analgesic properties. Dosage and Safety, As with any herbal remedy, the correct dosage is key. Dosages should be adjusted for children based on weight and age. Safety must always come first—parents should ensure they're using herbs that are safe for children and consult with healthcare professionals before beginning any new treatment. "The Book of Natural Medicine and Herbal Remedies," provides parents with a comprehensive guide to treating common childhood ailments with herbal remedies. This section covers various illnesses, appropriate herbs, preparation methods, dosages, and safety precautions to give parents the tools they need to support their children's health naturally.

Herbal Support for Growth and Development

Fostering Growth and Development with Herbal Support, As children grow, parents often seek natural ways to support their development. Certain herbs can provide nutritional support and promote overall well-being during these crucial years.

Nutritive Herbs Nettle (Urtica dioica): Nettle is rich in vitamins and minerals, including iron, which is essential for healthy blood and energy levels.

Oatstraw (Avena sativa): Oatstraw is another nutritive herb that supports nervous system health and can help with stress and anxiety, which can impact growth and development. Herbs for Bone Health Horsetail (Equisetum arvense): Horsetail contains silica, which is important for bone and connective tissue health.

Dandelion (Taraxacum officinale): The leaves are high in calcium and vitamin K, both vital for bone growth and strength. Dandelion can be eaten raw in salads or prepared as a tea.

Supporting Digestive Health Peppermint (Mentha piperita): A healthy digestive system is crucial for the absorption of nutrients necessary for growth. Peppermint can aid digestion and relieve digestive discomfort.

Ginger (Zingiber officinale): Ginger supports digestive health and can help with the absorption of nutrients. Herbs for Immune Support Astragalus **(Astragalus membranaceus):** Known for its immune-boosting properties, astragalus can help protect against common illnesses that can affect growth.

Echinacea (Echinacea spp.): As previously mentioned, Echinacea supports the immune system, which is essential for uninterrupted growth and development.

Cognitive Development Gotu Kola (Centella asiatica): Gotu Kola is believed to support brain health and may improve concentration and cognitive function.

Rosemary (Rosmarinus officinalis): Rosemary has been traditionally used to improve memory and concentration. Safety and Professional Guidance While these herbs are known for their supportive properties, it's critical to use them safely. Parents should consult with healthcare professionals to ensure these herbs are appropriate for their children's specific needs.

Herbal Care for Skin and Allergies

In-Depth Herbal Care for Skin and Allergies

Calendula (Calendula officinalis)

Uses: Calendula is a versatile herb that can be used to soothe various skin conditions such as eczema, diaper rash, and minor cuts or burns.

Preparation: For topical use, calendula can be infused in oil and applied directly to the skin or incorporated into creams and salves. Calendula tea can also be used as a wash for irritated skin areas.

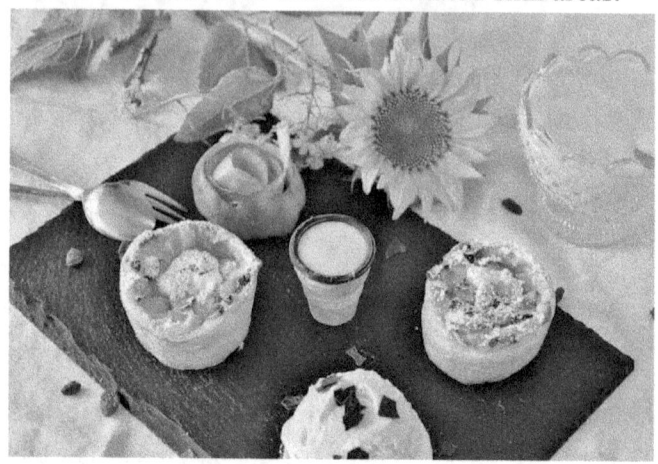

Chickweed (Stellaria media)

Uses: Chickweed is particularly effective for itchy and inflamed skin. It's gentle enough for use on sensitive skin and can provide relief from eczema and psoriasis.

Preparation: Chickweed can be made into a poultice by crushing fresh leaves and applying them to the affected area. It can also be included in creams or ointments for easier application.

Plantain (Plantago major)

Uses: Plantain is known for its quick relief of insect bites, stings, and allergic reactions on the skin. It can reduce swelling and soothe irritation.

Preparation: Fresh plantain leaves can be chewed or crushed to release their juices and then applied to the skin. Alternatively, plantain-infused oil or cream can be used.

Nettle (Urtica dioica)

Uses: Nettle's natural antihistamine properties make it a go-to herb for seasonal allergies. It can help alleviate symptoms like sneezing, itching, and runny nose.

Preparation: Nettle tea is a common preparation for allergy relief. Dried nettle leaves can also be encapsulated or made into a tincture.

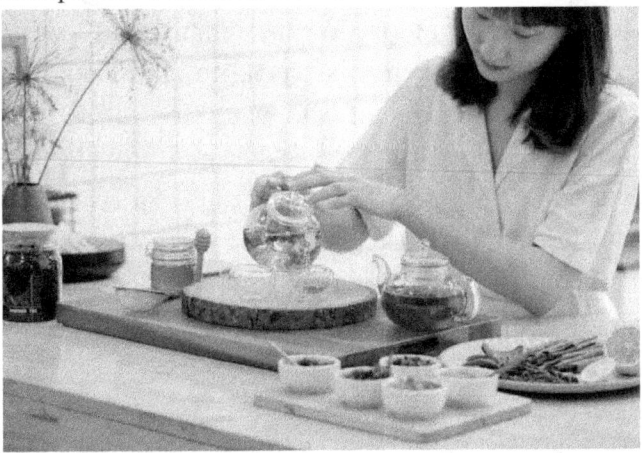

Eyebright (Euphrasia officinalis)

Uses: Eyebright is traditionally used to relieve eye irritation caused by allergies. It has astringent

properties that help reduce inflammation.
Preparation: Eyebright tea can be cooled and used as an eye compress. It's also available in tincture form, which can be diluted in water and used as an eye wash.

Licorice Root (Glycyrrhiza glabra)
Uses: Licorice root has soothing properties that are beneficial for treating allergic reactions. It's important to note that licorice should be used with caution due to its potent effects. Licorice root tea is one way to administer this herb. It can also be taken as a tincture or syrup but should always be under the guidance of a healthcare professional due to potential side effects.

Dosage Considerations When administering herbal remedies to children, it's crucial to adjust dosages based on their weight and age. Consult with a paediatric herbalist or healthcare provider to determine the appropriate dosage. Safety Tips, Always perform a patch test when using new topical treatments to ensure there's no allergic reaction. Monitor children closely when introducing new herbs into their regimen.

Chapter 10: Herbal Detox and Cleansing

Benefits of Detoxification

Detoxification aids in the optimal functioning of vital organs such as the liver, kidneys, and colon, which are instrumental in filtering and eliminating toxins from the body. By supporting these organs, detoxification can lead to better nutrient absorption, improved digestion, and a more robust immune system capable of fighting off infections. Additionally, it can contribute to healthier skin by aiding the body in expelling waste through sweat and sebum, leading to a clearer complexion and reduced acne.

Enhanced Mental Clarity: The accumulation of toxins in the body can impair brain function, resulting in symptoms like brain fog, memory issues, and a lack of focus. Detoxification helps clear these toxins from the bloodstream, which can improve blood flow to the brain and enhance cognitive functions such as concentration and memory retention.

Strengthened Immune System: A heavy toxic load can overburden the body's detoxifying organs, weakening the immune system's ability to fight off pathogens. By engaging in detoxification practices, we reduce this burden, allowing the immune system to recover and strengthen. This can lead to fewer illnesses and a better overall state of health.

Increased Energy Levels: Toxins can negatively impact metabolism and energy production within the body. By removing these toxins through detoxification, metabolic processes can become more efficient, leading to increased energy levels, reduced lethargy, and a greater sense of vitality.

Weight Management: Detoxification can support weight management by improving metabolic rate and aiding in the elimination of waste products. It may also help reset appetite regulation and reduce cravings for unhealthy foods, making it easier to maintain a healthy weight.

Relief from Digestive Issues: A detox can help rebalance the digestive system by removing waste products that may be causing bloating, constipation, or other gastrointestinal issues. This leads to improved gut health and regular bowel movements.

Healthier Skin: The skin is one of the primary organs involved in excreting toxins from the body. Detoxification practices support skin health by facilitating the removal of toxins through sweat glands, which can result in a clearer complexion and reduced incidence of skin disorders such as eczema or psoriasis.

Reduction in Aches and Fatigue: The presence of toxins in muscles and tissues can contribute to inflammation and pain. Detoxification helps alleviate these symptoms by reducing toxin levels in the body, which may lead to a decrease in chronic pain conditions, headaches, muscle stiffness, and overall fatigue.

Herbs for Liver Health

Milk Thistle (Silymarin): Milk thistle is perhaps the most well-known herb for liver health. The active compound, silymarin, is a complex mixture of flavonolignans, which are thought to contribute to its hepatoprotective and regenerative properties. Silymarin acts as an antioxidant, scavenging free radicals and stabilising cell membranes. It also stimulates protein synthesis, which aids in the regeneration of damaged liver cells. Clinical studies have suggested that milk thistle may be beneficial in treating liver diseases such as alcoholic hepatitis, cirrhosis, liver poisoning, and viral hepatitis.

Turmeric (Curcumin): Turmeric's bright yellow color comes from curcumin, a polyphenolic compound with strong antioxidant and anti-inflammatory properties. Curcumin has been shown to modulate several molecular targets involved in liver health, including enzymes, cytokines, and growth factors. It's been studied for its effects on liver fibrosis and its ability to enhance bile production, which helps the body rid itself of toxins.

Green Tea (Catechins): Green tea is rich in catechins, a type of natural phenol and antioxidant. Epigallocatechin gallate (EGCG) is the most abundant catechin in green tea and has been extensively studied for its liver-protective effects. EGCG has been shown to reduce liver inflammation and fat deposition in the liver, which can help prevent non-alcoholic fatty liver disease.

Dandelion Root: Dandelion root has a long history of use as a liver tonic in traditional herbal medicine. It contains sesquiterpene lactones, which are thought to stimulate digestion by increasing bile flow. This increased bile flow helps to break down fats and promote digestion while also helping the liver detoxify more efficiently.

Ginger: Ginger contains gingerol, a compound with powerful anti-inflammatory and antioxidant effects.

Gingerol has been shown to help protect against liver fibrosis by inhibiting the formation of scar tissue in the liver.

Garlic: Garlic is rich in sulfur-containing compounds such as allicin, which are believed to activate liver enzymes that help your body flush out toxins. Garlic also has high amounts of selenium, an essential micronutrient that has been shown to have hepatoprotective properties.

Ginseng: Ginseng has been used in traditional Chinese medicine for centuries for its numerous health benefits, including its ability to improve liver function. Ginsenosides, the active compounds in ginseng, have been shown to have anti-inflammatory effects that may be beneficial for liver health.

Licorice: Licorice contains glycyrrhizin, which has been shown to have antiviral properties against hepatitis C virus (HCV) and other forms of chronic hepatitis.

Astragalus: Astragalus is known for its immune-boosting properties and has been used traditionally to treat chronic hepatitis and as a complementary therapy for cancer patients undergoing chemotherapy or radiation therapy.

Artichoke: Artichoke leaves contain cynarin and silymarin, both of which have demonstrated hepatoprotective effects by enhancing bile production and protecting against toxins.

Schisandra: Schisandra berries are believed to protect the liver from poisons, prevent liver damage, and promote the growth of new liver cells. Burdock

Root: Burdock root is known for its blood-purifying properties and contains compounds that have been found to detoxify heavy metals from the blood, improving organ health including that of the liver.

Chicory Root: Chicory root boosts the body's systems related to detoxification due to its high inulin content, a type of soluble fibre that promotes digestive health and supports liver function. Yellow

Dock: Yellow dock root is traditionally used as a blood purifier and general detoxifier, especially for the liver.

Boldo: Boldo leaves contain boldine, an alkaloid that has been shown to protect against oxidative stress-induced damage in the liver.

Herbal Support for Kidney and Urinary Health

Herbal remedies have been used for centuries to support kidney and urinary health, offering natural ways to cleanse, protect, and improve the function of these vital systems. Here's a detailed exploration of some herbs that are particularly beneficial.

Dandelion: Known for its diuretic properties, dandelion can help increase urine production, aiding in the removal of waste products and excess fluids from the kidneys. It's also believed to support the elimination of kidney stones.

Parsley: Another diuretic herb, parsley can help flush out toxins from the kidneys and urinary tract. It's also rich in antioxidants, which may protect the kidneys from damage caused by free radicals.

Cranberries: Drinking cranberry juice is a well-known remedy for urinary tract infections (UTIs). Cranberries contain compounds that prevent bacteria from adhering to the urinary tract walls, reducing the risk of infections.

Nettle Leaf: Nettle has natural diuretic effects and is often used to promote kidney detoxification. It may also help in managing symptoms of benign prostatic hyperplasia (BPH), which can affect urinary flow.

Corn Silk: The silky threads of the corn plant have been traditionally used to treat bladder irritation and reduce symptoms of UTIs. They may also help in preventing kidney stone formation.

Clove: With potent antimicrobial properties, clove bud can be useful in treating acute bladder infections. It's also an anti-inflammatory agent, which can soothe the urinary tract.

Couchgrass: Traditionally used for bladder and kidney ailments, couchgrass acts as a gentle diuretic and has soothing properties that can help with UTIs and cystitis.

Cleavers: This herb is known to support lymphatic drainage and urinary health. It's often used to treat urinary problems such as cystitis and urethritis. Remember, while these herbs offer many potential benefits, it's crucial to consult with a healthcare professional before using them, especially if you have existing kidney problems or are taking medications. Each herb should be understood in-depth for its properties, dosage, and contraindications to ensure safe and effective use in promoting kidney and urinary health.

Detoxifying Teas and Tonics

Detoxifying teas and tonics are a cornerstone of natural medicine, offering a gentle yet effective way to cleanse the body and support overall health. Here's an in-depth look at some of the most beneficial detoxifying teas and tonics.

Birch Tea: Birch leaves are known for their diuretic and depurative properties. They help eliminate waste products from the body and support kidney function, making birch tea an excellent choice for a detoxifying regimen.

Horsetail Tea: This herb is not only a diuretic but also rich in minerals. It's known for its astringent and hemostatic properties, which can help tone the urinary tract and stop bleeding, aiding in the detoxification process.

Juniper Tea: Juniper berries have a tonic effect on the body and are particularly beneficial for the urinary system. They also have diuretic properties, helping to cleanse the kidneys and bladder.

Sage Tea: Sage is a versatile herb with diuretic, tonic, stimulating, and expectorant properties. It can help detoxify the body by promoting sweating and supporting liver function.

Elderberry Tea: Known for its immune-boosting effects, elderberry also has diuretic, anti-inflammatory, and expectorant properties, making it a great addition to any detox tea blend.

Dandelion Root Tea: As mentioned earlier, dandelion root is excellent for kidney health and acts as a natural diuretic. It supports liver function as well, which is crucial for detoxification.

Fennel Seed Tea: Fennel seeds are known for their ability to aid digestion and relieve bloating. They also have diuretic properties that help in flushing out toxins from the body.

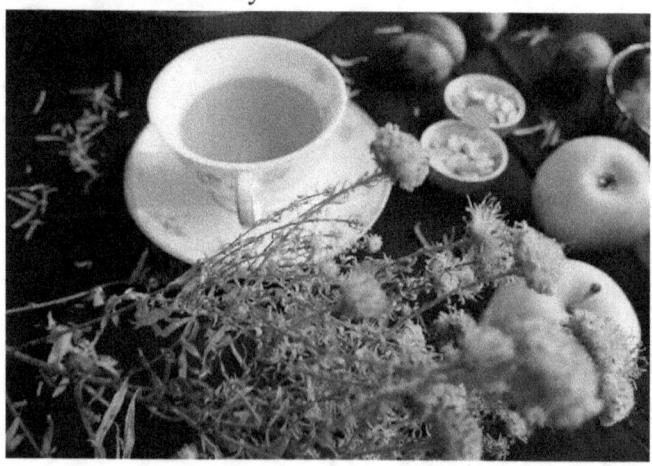

Holy Basil (Tulsi) Tea: This adaptogenic herb helps the body respond to stress and supports natural detoxification processes.

Licorice Root Tea: Licorice root is another powerful detoxifier that supports liver health. However, it should be used with caution, especially those who are pregnant or lactating. When creating detoxifying teas or tonics, it's essential to consider the specific needs of your body and any health conditions you may have.

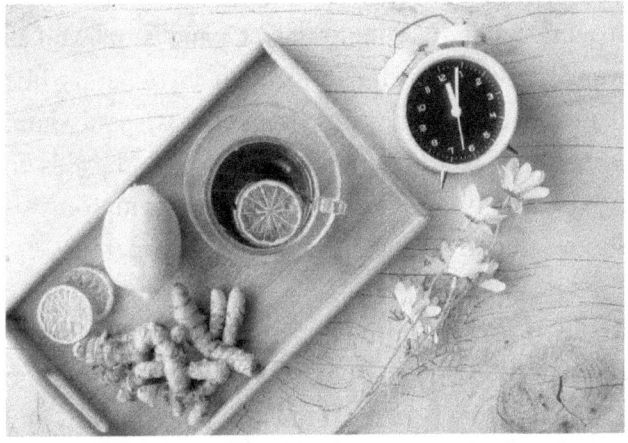

Always consult with a healthcare professional before starting any new herbal regimen, especially if you have existing health concerns or are taking medications. These teas can be enjoyed on their own or blended together for a synergistic effect. Incorporating these into your daily routine can provide a soothing experience while contributing to your body's natural cleansing processes.

Chapter 11: Herbal Nutrition

Nutrient-Rich Herbs

Nutrient-rich herbs are a treasure trove of vitamins and minerals that can significantly contribute to our daily nutritional intake. Here's an in-depth look at some of the most nutrient-dense herbs and their benefits.

Nettle (Urtica dioica): Nettle is a powerhouse of nutrients, including vitamins A, C, and K, as well as several B vitamins. It is also rich in minerals like calcium, iron, magnesium, phosphorus, potassium, and sodium. Nettle supports kidney health, aids in detoxification, and can help alleviate symptoms of allergies due to its anti-inflammatory properties.

Parsley (Petroselinum crispum): Parsley is not just a garnish; it's a nutritional powerhouse. It's high in vitamin K, which is essential for bone health, and vitamin C, a powerful antioxidant. Parsley also contains flavonoids that have been shown to have antioxidant properties.

Dandelion (Taraxacum officinale): As previously mentioned, dandelion is rich in vitamins A, C, and K. It also contains vitamin E and small amounts of other B vitamins. Alfalfa (Medicago sativa): Alfalfa leaves are rich in vitamins A, C, E, and K4. They also contain calcium, potassium, phosphorus, and iron. Alfalfa has been traditionally used to support kidney health and digestion.

Spirulina (Arthrospira platensis): Although not a herb in the traditional sense, spirulina is a blue-green algae that is incredibly nutrient-dense. It's a complete protein source and contains B vitamins, beta-carotene, vitamin E, manganese, zinc, copper, iron, selenium, and gamma-linolenic acid (an essential fatty acid).

Chlorella (Chlorella vulgaris): Like spirulina, chlorella is a type of algae that offers a wealth of nutrients. It's high in protein and omega-3 fatty acids and contains a range of vitamins and minerals. Incorporating these nutrient-rich herbs into your diet can be done in various ways—fresh or dried in culinary dishes, as herbal teas or infusions, or even as supplements in powder or capsule form.

They offer an array of health benefits from boosting the immune system to reducing inflammation and supporting detoxification processes. Always ensure you're sourcing your herbs from reputable suppliers to avoid contamination with pesticides or heavy metals. And remember to consult with a healthcare professional before starting any new supplement regimen.

Incorporating Herbs into Daily Diet

Incorporating herbs into your daily diet is a delightful way to boost both flavour and nutrition. Here are some practical tips to seamlessly integrate herbs into your meals.

1. Fresh Herbs in Salads: Toss fresh herbs like basil, cilantro, parsley, or mint into your salads. They add a burst of flavour and increase the nutritional value with their vitamins and minerals.

2. Herbs as Garnishes: Sprinkle chopped herbs over your finished dishes. Not only do they add a pop of colour and flavour, but they also provide health benefits. For example, garnishing with dill can aid digestion.

3. Smoothie Boosters: Add herbs like parsley or cilantro to your smoothies for a nutrient kick. They blend well with fruits and vegetables, enhancing the taste and upping the health quotient.

4. Seasoning with Herbs: Use dried or fresh herbs to season your dishes. They can replace salt in many recipes, helping to reduce sodium intake while adding depth to the flavor profile.

5. Herbal Teas: Brew teas from fresh or dried herbs like chamomile, peppermint, or lemon balm. These teas can be calming and aid in digestion or sleep.

6. Cooking with Herbs: Incorporate herbs into your cooking process. Add rosemary to roast meats, stir basil into pasta sauces, or mix cilantro into rice dishes.

7. Herb-Infused Oils and Vinegars: Create your own herb-infused oils and vinegars by steeping herbs in them. These can be used in dressings, marinades, or as a drizzle over cooked dishes.

8. Baking with Herbs: Herbs can be added to breads, scones, and other baked goods for an unexpected twist of flavour.

Remember that while it's generally safe to consume herbs daily, it's important to do so in moderation as excessive intake can be toxic1. Always store fresh herbs properly to maintain their flavor and nutritional benefits.

173

Herbal Supplements and Powders

Herbal supplements and powders are derived from plants whose parts have been used for medicinal purposes due to their healing properties. Unlike pharmaceutical drugs, herbal supplements are not highly regulated, which means it's essential to choose high-quality products from trusted sources.

Benefits and Uses:
1. Nutritional Boost: Many herbs are rich in vitamins, minerals, and antioxidants, which can help fill nutritional gaps in the diet. For example, nettle is high in iron, making it beneficial for individuals with anaemia.

2. Targeted Health Support: Specific herbs address particular health concerns. For instance, saw palmetto is often used to support prostate health, while echinacea is known for its immune-boosting properties.

3. Holistic Well-being: Herbs like ashwagandha and holy basil are adaptogens, which means they help the body resist stressors of all kinds, whether physical, chemical or biological.

4. Choosing Quality Supplements: Standardisation: Look for supplements that mention "standardised extract" on the label, which indicates a consistent level of active ingredients.

5. Certifications: Certifications from organizations like the U.S. Pharmacopeia (USP), NSF International, or ConsumerLab.com can provide assurance of quality.

6. Whole Herb vs. Extract: Decide whether you want a whole herb supplement, which contains all parts of the plant, or an extract, which may be more potent and targeted.

Safety Considerations:
Interactions with Medications: Some herbs can interact with prescription medications by enhancing or inhibiting their effects.

Side Effects:
While herbs are natural, they can still cause side effects or allergic reactions in some individuals.

Incorporating into Diet:
1. Teas and Infusions: Herbal teas are a simple way to enjoy the benefits of herbs. Infusions can be made by steeping herbs in hot water to extract their active compounds.

2. Cooking: Powders can be added to soups, stews, smoothies, or baked goods. Turmeric powder is commonly used in cooking for its anti-inflammatory properties.

3. Capsules and Tablets: These are convenient for those who prefer not to taste the herb or want a precise dosage.

Cooking with Herbs

Cooking with herbs is a delightful way to add depth and complexity to your dishes. Here's a comprehensive guide to using herbs in the kitchen.

1. Fresh vs. Dried Herbs: Fresh herbs offer a brighter flavour and are best added towards the end of cooking to preserve their essence. Dried herbs, on the other hand, have a more concentrated flavour and should be added during the cooking process to allow their flavours to meld into the dish.

2. Preparing Fresh Herbs: Wash and pat them dry before use. Chop finely or crush gently to release their flavours. Some herbs, like basil, can be torn by hand to prevent bruising.

3. Flavour Pairings: Match herbs with complementary foods. For example, rosemary pairs well with roasted meats, while cilantro complements spicy dishes.

4. Cooking Techniques: Infusing: Heat herbs with unsalted butter or oils to draw out their aromatic oils.
i. Garnishing: Use fresh herbs as a garnish to add a pop of flavour and colour.
ii. Marinating: Incorporate herbs into marinades for meats or vegetables to infuse them with flavour.

5. Quantity: Be mindful of the amount – too little won't add enough flavour, but too much can overpower a dish.

6. Preservation: To maintain the potency of herbs: Freezing: Freeze fresh herbs in ice cube trays with water or oil.
i. Drying: Hang bunches of fresh herbs upside down in a warm, dry place until completely dry.

7. Storage: Store fresh herbs in the refrigerator wrapped in a damp paper towel or standing upright in a glass of water. Dried herbs should be kept in a cool, dark place in an airtight container.

8. Experimentation: Don't be afraid to experiment with different herb combinations or using them in unexpected ways, like adding mint to salads or thyme to desserts.

Chapter 12: Herbal Remedies for Physical Fitness

Pre-Workout Herbs

Pre-workout herbs can offer a wide range of benefits to enhance your workout experience. Here's a detailed explanation of how these herbs can support your fitness goals.

1. Energy Boost: Herbs like green tea extract, coffee, yohimbe, and guarana contain natural stimulants that can increase alertness and energy levels, helping you feel more energized during your workout session.

2. Enhanced Focus: Certain herbs improve mental clarity and focus, which is crucial for maintaining proper form and staying motivated throughout your exercise routine. Yerba Mate, for example, is known to boost mental focus while also enhancing physical performance.

3. Improved Cardiovascular Function: Herbs such as Green Tea have been studied for their ability to support the cardiovascular system, which is essential for endurance and stamina during workouts.

4. Better Anaerobic Performance: Ingredients like carnitine and beta-alanine found in some herbal supplements can enhance anaerobic performance, allowing you to train harder and longer.

5. Recovery Support: Herbs can also aid in recovery post-workout. BCAAs (Branched-Chain Amino Acids) and glutamine are compounds that help reduce muscle soreness and boost recovery, so you're ready for your next session sooner.

6. Anti-Inflammatory Properties: Turmeric, for instance, promotes healthy joint function and mobility by supporting the body's inflammatory response, which can be particularly beneficial after intense workouts.

7. Adaptogenic Effects: Adaptogens like Ashwagandha and Rhodiola Rosea help the body adapt to stress and can improve energy utilization, reduce inflammation, and support overall athletic performance.

How They Work: These herbs work by various

mechanisms: Stimulating the Central Nervous **System:** To increase alertness and reduce the perception of effort. Supporting Metabolic **Processes:** That produce energy at the cellular level.

Enhancing Oxygen Utilization: To improve endurance.

Reducing Inflammation: To aid in recovery and reduce pain. incorporating these herbs into your pre-workout routine, either through teas, supplements, or powders, you can naturally enhance your physical capabilities and recovery process. Always ensure to use these herbs responsibly and consult with a healthcare provider to avoid any potential interactions with medications or health conditions.

Herbs for Muscle Recovery

Herbs can be a natural and effective way to support muscle recovery after intense physical activity. Here's a detailed explanation of some herbs known for their recovery benefits.

1. Turmeric (Curcumin): Contains curcumin, a compound with strong anti-inflammatory properties that can help reduce muscle pain and soreness after exercise.

2. Ashwagandha: An adaptogen that helps the body manage stress and can boost muscle recovery by reducing inflammation and improving sleep quality, which is crucial for muscle repair.

3. Rhodiola Rosea: Another adaptogen known to improve physical performance and reduce recovery time by balancing the body's stress response system.

4. Beetroot: Rich in nitrates, beetroot can enhance blood flow to muscles, improving oxygen delivery and aiding in recovery.

5. Tongkat Ali: May increase muscle strength and size by affecting hormone levels that contribute to muscle growth and recovery.

6. Capsaicin: Found in chili peppers, capsaicin can act as a natural pain reliever and may help reduce muscle soreness.

7. Lemongrass: Its anti-inflammatory properties can help soothe sore muscles and improve recovery times.

8. Ginseng: Can enhance physical endurance and post-exercise recovery by modulating the immune response and reducing oxidative stress.

9. Maca: Known for its energy-boosting properties, maca can also support muscle growth and recovery by providing essential vitamins and minerals

How They Work:

Reducing Inflammation: Many of these herbs contain compounds that help reduce inflammation, which is a common cause of muscle soreness.

1. Improving Circulation: Herbs like beetroot improve blood flow, which helps remove waste products from muscles more efficiently.

2. Balancing Stress Hormones: Adaptogens like ashwagandha and rhodiola help regulate cortisol levels, which can otherwise impede recovery.

3. Pain Relief: Some herbs have analgesic properties that can alleviate the discomfort associated with muscle recovery.

How to Use Them:

1. Supplements: Capsules or tablets containing these herbs can be taken according to the recommended dosage.

2. Teas: Herbal teas made from these plants can be consumed post-workout for their soothing effects.

Topical Applications:

Some herbs are available in creams or gels that can be applied directly to sore muscles. As with any supplement.

it's important to consult with a healthcare provider before incorporating these herbs into your routine, especially if you have health conditions or are taking other medications.

Enhancing Endurance with Herbs

Herbs have been used for centuries to enhance physical performance and endurance. Their wide-ranging benefits can be attributed to their diverse active compounds that support various physiological functions. Here's a comprehensive overview.

1. Physiological Benefits: Oxygen Efficiency: Herbs like rhodiola and cordyceps have been shown to improve the body's oxygen utilization. Rhodiola increases the red blood cell count, which is crucial for transporting oxygen to muscles, while cordyceps improves lung function and oxygen uptake.

2. Blood Flow: Ginkgo biloba and hawthorn have been found to enhance blood flow. Ginkgo does this by dilating blood vessels and reducing blood viscosity, whereas hawthorn improves coronary artery blood flow, enhancing the oxygen supply to the heart muscle.

3. Hormonal Balance: Herbs such as maca root and ashwagandha can influence hormone profiles. Maca root contains compounds that may help balance hormones and improve energy levels, while ashwagandha has been shown to increase testosterone levels in men, leading to improved muscle mass and endurance.

Stress Adaptation: Adaptogens like ashwagandha and eleuthero help the body adapt to physical stress by modulating the release of stress hormones from the adrenal glands. This can lead to improved performance and endurance.

Types of Herbs and Their Applications:

1. Adaptogenic Herbs: These herbs help the body resist physical, chemical, and biological stressors. Ashwagandha, for example, has been shown to improve endurance by increasing nitric oxide production, which helps in vasodilation and improves blood flow.

2. Cardiovascular Support Herbs: Hawthorn is particularly beneficial for cardiovascular health as it can increase cardiac output by improving heart muscle contractions. Ginkgo biloba also supports cardiovascular function by improving circulation.

3. Energy-Boosting Herbs: Green tea contains caffeine, which can enhance physical performance by increasing alertness and energy levels. Cordyceps is known for boosting mitochondrial function, which plays a key role in energy production.

Incorporating Herbs into Your Routine:

1. Supplementation: Herbal supplements should be taken according to recommended dosages on product labels or as advised by a healthcare provider.

2. Dietary Inclusion: Some herbs can be included in meals; for instance, powdered maca root can be added to smoothies or oatmeal for an energy boost.

3. Herbal Teas: Drinking herbal teas is a convenient way to consume herbs that support endurance. For example, ginseng tea can be consumed before workouts for an energy lift.

Safety and Precautions:

Quality of Herbs: It's important to source high-quality herbs that are free from contaminants. **Interactions with Medications:** Be cautious of potential interactions between herbs and medications you may be taking.

Allergies and Sensitivities: Always be aware of personal allergies or sensitivities to specific herbs.

Herbal Solutions for Inflammation

Herbal remedies have been used for centuries to reduce inflammation, which is the body's natural response to injury or infection. Here's a detailed look at some herbs with anti-inflammatory properties.

1. Turmeric (Curcuma longa): Active Compound: Curcumin is the main active compound in turmeric, responsible for its bright yellow colour and many of its health benefits.
Mechanism: Curcumin has been shown to block NF-kB, a molecule that travels into the nuclei of cells and turns on genes related to inflammation.

2.. Studies: Numerous studies have demonstrated curcumin's ability to reduce biomarkers of inflammation in the blood. A review published in the Journal of Medicinal Food suggests that curcumin can help manage exercise-induced inflammation and muscle soreness, thus enhancing recovery and subsequent performance in active people.

3. **Ginger (Zingiber officinale):** Active Compounds: Gingerol is the main bioactive compound in ginger, responsible for much of its medicinal properties.
Mechanism: Gingerol has powerful anti-inflammatory and antioxidant effects. According to a study published in the International Journal of Preventive Medicine, ginger supplementation significantly reduced inflammatory markers in the blood.
Traditional Use:
Ginger has been used for thousands of years to aid digestion, reduce nausea, and help fight the flu and common cold.

4. **Green Tea (Camellia sinensis):**
Active Compounds: The most powerful compound in green tea is epigallocatechin gallate (EGCG), which has been studied to treat various diseases and may be one of the main reasons green tea has such powerful medicinal properties.
Mechanism: EGCG has been found to reduce inflammation by lowering cytokine production and damage to the fatty acids in your cells.
Studies: A study published in the Journal of Advanced Research indicates that green tea can

reduce inflammation markers and help prevent certain chronic diseases associated with inflammation.

2. Rosemary (Rosmarinus officinalis):

Active Compounds: The active components in rosemary are antioxidant compounds such as rosmarinic acid and carnosic acid.

Mechanism: These compounds have been shown to suppress inflammatory responses by altering the synthesis of inflammatory mediators such as prostaglandins.

Traditional Use: Rosemary has been used traditionally for improving memory, aiding digestion, and as a natural preservative due to its antioxidant properties.

5. Cinnamon (Cinnamomum verum): Active Compounds: Cinnamaldehyde is one of the most active components of cinnamon and gives it its distinctive smell and flavour.

Mechanism: Cinnamaldehyde inhibits the activation of inflammatory pathways within blood cells and tissues, helping to prevent inflammation. **Studies:** Research published in Evidence-Based Complementary and Alternative Medicine found that cinnamon extracts have potential anti-inflammatory properties.

6. Garlic (Allium sativum): Active Compounds: Garlic contains diallyl disulfide, an anti-inflammatory compound that limits the effects of pro-inflammatory cytokines.

Mechanism: Garlic oil has been shown to protect against cartilage damage from arthritis.

Traditional Use: Garlic has been used throughout history for its medicinal properties, with records indicating its use for cardiovascular health, prevention of colds, and more.

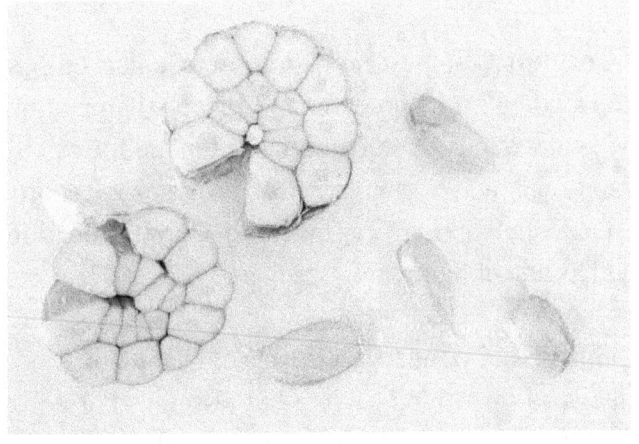

Chapter 13: Herbal Remedies for Beauty and Skincare

Natural Skincare Ingredients

Natural ingredients are increasingly popular in skincare due to their gentle nature and potent benefits. Here's a detailed look at some natural skincare ingredients.

1. Coconut Oil: Beyond hydration, coconut oil has been studied for its potential to reduce inflammation and heal wounds. A study published in the Journal of Traditional and Complementary Medicine reports that coconut oil can improve skin barrier function and has anti-inflammatory properties.

2. Gotu Kola (Centella asiatica): This plant is not only good for wound healing but also for improving skin elasticity and reducing stretch marks. Research in the Journal of Ethnopharmacology highlights its ability to stimulate collagen production and mitigate the formation of stretch marks.

3. Green Tea: The polyphenols in green tea, particularly EGCG, have been shown to protect against UV radiation and improve skin hydration. A study in the Journal of Nutrition found that green tea polyphenols can help prevent skin disorders associated with exposure to UV radiation.

4. **Oatmeal:** Oatmeal contains compounds called avenanthramides that have anti-inflammatory and antioxidant properties. Clinical studies, such as one published in the Journal of Drugs in Dermatology, have demonstrated oatmeal's effectiveness in treating dry, itchy, and atopic skin.

4. **Shea Butter:** Shea butter is rich in triterpenes, which have been shown to reduce inflammation. A study in the American Journal of Life Sciences suggests that shea butter can improve skin moisture and elasticity.

5. **Soy:** Soy's isoflavones have been studied for their anti-aging effects on the skin. The Journal of Drugs in Dermatology published a study indicating that soy isoflavones can improve skin thickness and elasticity.

6. **Tea Tree Oil:** Known for its antimicrobial properties, tea tree oil has been proven effective against acne-causing bacteria. The Australasian Journal of Dermatology published a study showing that a 5% tea tree oil solution can treat mild to moderate acne as effectively as 5% benzoyl

peroxide. These natural ingredients are backed by scientific research demonstrating their efficacy in skincare. They offer a range of benefits from moisturizing and anti-inflammatory effects to anti-aging and antimicrobial actions. When using these ingredients, it's important to consider your specific skin needs and consult with a dermatologist if you have any concerns or conditions.

Herbal Hair Care

Herbal hair care involves using natural herbs and plants to nourish, strengthen, and protect the hair. Here are some key herbal ingredients and their benefits for hair care.

1. Aloe Vera: Known for its hydrating properties, aloe vera can soothe the scalp and condition the hair. It's rich in vitamins A, C, and E, which contribute to cell turnover and promote healthy hair growth. Amla (Indian Gooseberry): Amla is high in vitamin C and antioxidants.

2. Basil: This herb stimulates hair follicles, enhances blood circulation in the scalp, and promotes hair growth.

3. Bhringraj (Eclipta alba): Often referred to as the "king of herbs" for hair growth, bhringraj is believed to rejuvenate the hair, prevent baldness, and treat dandruff and dry scalp.

4. Burdock Root: Rich in fatty acids, burdock root can improve scalp health by reducing inflammation and dandruff. It also promotes natural hair growth by improving blood circulation to the hair follicles.

5. Saw Palmetto: This herb is known for its ability to combat hair loss. It's believed to block the enzyme that converts testosterone into DHT, a molecule associated with male pattern baldness.

6. Wheat Germ: Packed with vitamins and minerals, wheat germ helps nourish the hair follicles. It's particularly beneficial for promoting stronger, healthier hair.

7. Oat Extract: Oat extract soothes the scalp and enhances hair texture. It makes the hair more manageable and can help treat dryness and itchiness.

When using these herbs for hair care:

1. Infusions: Make an infusion by steeping herbs in hot water to create a rinse or add to shampoos.

2. Oils: Use herbal oils to massage the scalp, which can stimulate blood flow and promote hair growth.

3. Masks: Create a paste or mask with powdered herbs for deep conditioning treatments.

4. Dietary Supplements: Some herbs can be taken internally as supplements to support overall health, which reflects in hair quality. Herbal ingredients offer a natural approach to maintaining healthy hair. They can be used in various forms such as oils, masks, shampoos, or even dietary supplements.

Anti-Aging Herbal Remedies

For a more in-depth understanding of anti-aging herbal remedies, let's explore some of the top herbs and their specific benefits.

1. Ginseng: Ginseng is highly regarded for its anti-aging properties. It contains compounds known as ginsenosides, which have been shown to counteract oxidative stress and enhance cellular health. Ginseng can be consumed as tea, taken in capsule form, or applied topically in creams.

2. Turmeric: The active compound in turmeric, curcumin, has strong antioxidant properties that protect cells from damage. It's also known for its ability to modulate inflammation, which is a key factor in ageing. Turmeric can be added to food, taken as a supplement, or used in topical skin treatments.

3. Ginkgo Biloba: Ginkgo is famous for its neuroprotective effects. It improves blood flow to the brain and has antioxidant properties that may protect against age-related cognitive decline. Ginkgo can be taken as a supplement or tea.

4. Milk Thistle: Silymarin, found in milk thistle, is an antioxidant that may protect the liver from toxins and help regenerate liver cells. Milk thistle supplements are commonly available.

5. Goji Berries: These berries are rich in antioxidants, particularly carotenoids like zeaxanthin, which protect the eyes and skin from damage. Goji berries can be eaten raw, dried, or as a juice.

5. Reishi Mushrooms: Reishi contains compounds that may boost the immune system and have anti-cancer properties. They can be consumed as tea, extracts, or supplements.

6. Horsetail: Horsetail's high silica content helps maintain skin elasticity and improve the condition of hair and nails. It can be taken as a tea or supplement or used in hair rinses.

DIY Herbal Beauty Recipes

Creating your own herbal beauty products can be a fun and natural way to enhance your beauty routine. Here are some DIY herbal beauty recipes you can try at home.

1. Lavender Body Scrub

Ingredients:
1 cup granulated sugar
1/4 cup coconut oil
10 drops lavender essential oil
2 tablespoons dried lavender flowers (optional)

Instructions:
1: Combine the sugar and coconut oil in a bowl and mix well.
2. Add the lavender essential oil and mix well.
3. If desired, stir in the dried lavender flowers.
4. Gently rub the scrub onto your skin in a circular motion and rinse off with warm water.

2. Rosemary Hair Rinse

Ingredients:
1 cup water

1/2 onion; 4 garlic cloves, peeled; 2 tablespoons fresh rosemary leaves or 1 tablespoon dried rosemary; 1 lemon, zest of; 1 tablespoon
1 tablespoon apple cider vinegar

Instructions:
1. Bring the water to a boil, then remove from heat.
2. Add the rosemary leaves and let them steep for 20-30 minutes.
3. Strain the rosemary infusion and allow it to cool.
4. Add the apple cider vinegar and mix well.
5. After shampooing your hair, pour the rosemary hair rinse over your hair, making sure to cover the entire scalp and strands.
6. Leave it on for 5-10 minutes, then rinse with cool water.

4. Green Tea Facial Toner

Ingredients:
1 cup brewed green tea (cooled)
1 tablespoon witch hazel
2 drops tea tree essential oil (optional)

Instructions:
1. Combine the brewed green tea, witch hazel, and tea tree essential oil (if using) in a small spray bottle.
2. Shake well to mix the ingredients.

3. After cleansing your face, spray the toner onto a cotton pad and gently swipe it over your face, avoiding the eye area.

5. Rose and Oatmeal Bath Soak

Ingredients:
1 cup rolled oats
1/2 cup dried rose petals
1/4 cup powdered milk
10 drops rose essential oil (optional)

Instructions:
1. Place the rolled oats in a blender or food processor and pulse until they reach a fine consistency.
2. Combine the ground oats, dried rose petals, powdered milk, and rose essential oil (if using) in a mixing bowl.
3. Transfer the mixture to an airtight container or jar.
4. To use, add 1/2 cup of the bath soak to warm bathwater and enjoy a relaxing, skin-soothing bath.

6. Peppermint Foot Soak

Ingredients:
1/2 cup Epsom salt
2 tablespoons dried peppermint leaves
5 drops peppermint essential oil

Instructions:

1. In a medium-sized bowl, combine the Epsom salt and dried peppermint leaves.
2. Add the peppermint essential oil and mix well.
3. Fill a basin with warm water and add the peppermint foot soak mixture.
4. Soak your feet for 10-15 minutes to refresh and revitalise tired feet.

always patch test any new beauty product on a small area of skin before using it more extensively to ensure you don't have any adverse reactions. Enjoy creating and using these natural, herbal beauty recipes.

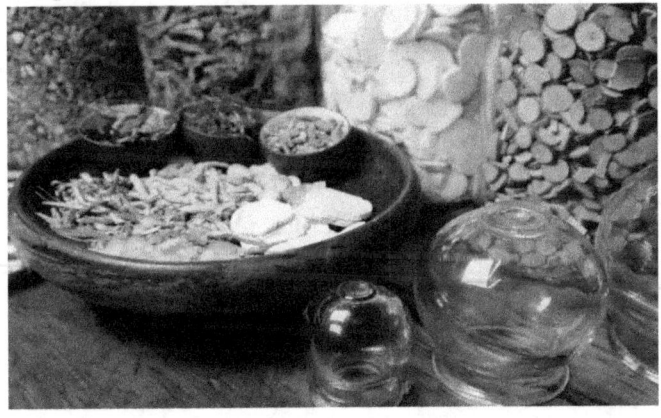

Chapter 14: Integrating Herbs into Daily Life

Creating a Home Apothecary

Creating a home apothecary is a rewarding and educational journey that combines aspects of herbalism, natural wellness, and self-sufficiency. This comprehensive guide will help you establish a well-organised and functional home apothecary tailored to your specific needs and interests.

1. Selecting the Right Space: Choose a dedicated area in your home that is dry, cool, and away from direct sunlight to preserve the quality of your herbal preparations and extend their shelf life.

i. Ensure the space is free from heat sources and not subject to drastic temperature changes, which can negatively impact the potency of your herbs.

ii. Consider factors like storage capacity, work surfaces, and ventilation when selecting your apothecary space.

2. Starting with Essential Herbs: Begin by stocking versatile, easy-to-find herbs that have multiple applications, such as chamomile, peppermint, lavender, and calendula.

i. As you gain experience and knowledge, expand your collection to include more specialised herbs that cater to specific health concerns or interests.

ii. Opt for high-quality herbs from reputable sources, either through online suppliers, local apothecaries, or by growing your own herbs at home.

3. Gathering Supplies: Invest in a variety of storage containers, such as glass jars of various sizes for dried herbs, and amber bottles for storing tinctures and other light-sensitive preparations.

i. Acquire essential tools, like mortars and pestles for grinding herbs, measuring spoons for accurate dosing, and funnels for bottling tinctures and other liquids.

ii. Optional equipment may include a scale for weighing herbs, a double boiler for oil infusions, and cheesecloth or muslin for straining.

4. Organising Your Apothecary: Implement a clear labelling system that includes the herb's name, date of acquisition or preparation, and any additional information relevant to the specific herb or preparation.

i. Arrange herbs alphabetically, by their medicinal properties, or by their intended use for easy access and reference.

ii. Regularly inventory your stock to track usage and identify any items that need replenishing or replacing.

5. Creating Herbal Remedies: Start with basic herbal preparations, such as teas, tinctures, salves, and infused oils, following reliable recipes and safety guidelines.
i. Experiment with different methods and techniques as your knowledge and confidence grow, documenting your processes and results for future reference.
ii. Begin with small batches to ensure freshness and minimise waste, adjusting quantities as you become more experienced.

6. Educating Yourself: Develop a strong foundation in herbalism by reading books, taking online courses, attending workshops, or participating in local herbalist communities.
i. Learn about individual herbs' properties, potential interactions, and appropriate dosage for safe and effective use.
ii. Stay up-to-date on the latest research and practices in herbal medicine to continually improve your home apothecary.

7. Maintaining Your Apothecary: Regularly assess the quality of your herbs and preparations, discarding any items that show signs of spoilage, mould, or diminished potency.

i. Keep your workspace clean and organized to maintain the integrity of your herbal products and facilitate an efficient workflow.

ii. Continuously expand your knowledge and skills by exploring new herbs, remedies, and techniques, keeping your home apothecary dynamic and evolving.

following these guidelines and actively engaging in the world of herbalism, you can create a thriving home apothecary that empowers you to take charge of your health and wellbeing while enjoying the many benefits that plants and natural remedies have to offer.

Herbal Self-Care Practices

Herbal self-care practices offer a holistic approach to wellbeing, leveraging the natural healing properties of plants to nourish and rejuvenate the body, mind, and spirit. By incorporating herbs into daily routines, individuals can support their overall health and foster a deeper connection with nature. Here's a more detailed exploration of some popular herbal self-care practices.

1. Herbal Infusions: Nutrient-rich herbs like nettle, oatstraw, or red clover can be steeped in hot water to create mineral-rich infusions that promote overall well-being. These infusions provide essential vitamins and minerals, as well as support for specific body systems.

2. Herbal Baths: Adding soothing herbs like lavender, chamomile, or rose petals to bathwater can create a calming and skin-soothing experience. This practice not only offers relaxation but can also help with skin inflammation, irritation, and stress relief.

3. Aromatherapy: Diffusing essential oils derived from herbs like peppermint, eucalyptus, or lemon balm can help enhance mood, alleviate stress, and purify the air. The aromatic compounds in these herbs can impact the limbic system, influencing emotions and memory.

4. Herbal Teas: Sipping on herbal teas, particularly those made from calming herbs such as lemon balm, passionflower, or valerian root, can aid in stress reduction and improved sleep quality. These herbs contain compounds that promote relaxation and support the body's natural sleep mechanisms.

5. Topical Herbal Remedies: Applying salves or balms made with skin-healing herbs like calendula, comfrey, or plantain can help soothe and heal a variety of skin conditions. The anti-inflammatory, antimicrobial, and analgesic properties of these herbs provide natural relief for various skin issues.

6. Herbal Smoke Cleansing: Burning dried herbs such as sage, cedar, or sweetgrass in a process known as "smudging" can cleanse the energy of a space and promote a sense of peace and tranquility. This practice has roots in traditional indigenous ceremonies and is often used to clear negative energy and create a more harmonious environment.

7. Herbal Cooking: Incorporating fresh or dried culinary herbs, like basil, thyme, or rosemary, into meals can enhance flavor while also providing additional health benefits. These herbs contain various antioxidant, antimicrobial, and anti-inflammatory compounds that support overall wellness.

8. Herbal Honey: Infusing honey with herbs like ginger, cinnamon, or thyme can create a delicious treat with added medicinal properties. This sweet concoction can help soothe sore throats, alleviate coughs, and support immune function. to source herbs sustainably and consult with a healthcare provider before starting any new herbal regimen, particularly if you have existing health conditions or are taking medications. Researching proper preparation and dosage is crucial to ensure the safe and effective use of herbal remedies.

Herbal Remedies for Pets

Herbal remedies can be used for pets as a natural approach to support their overall health and well-being. However, it's important to consult with a veterinarian before administering any herbal remedies to your pets, as some herbs may be toxic or interact with medications. Here are some examples of herbal remedies that can be beneficial for pets.

1. Chamomile (Matricaria chamomilla): Chamomile has soothing properties that can help reduce anxiety and promote relaxation in pets. It can be administered as a tea or a diluted essential oil.

2. Echinacea (Echinacea purpurea): Echinacea is known for its immune-boosting properties and can help support pets' immune systems, especially during times of stress or illness. It is usually administered as a tincture or in capsule form.

3. Milk Thistle (Silybum marianum): Milk thistle is a powerful antioxidant that can support liver function and detoxification in pets. It can be given as a tincture or in capsule form.

4. Peppermint (Mentha piperita): Peppermint can help alleviate digestive issues in pets, such as gas, bloating, and nausea. It can be administered as a tea, diluted essential oil, or in capsule form.

5. Valerian (Valeriana officinalis): Valerian has calming properties that can help reduce anxiety and promote relaxation in pets. It is usually administered as a tincture, tea, or in capsule form.

6. Dandelion (Taraxacum officinale): Dandelion can support kidney function and aid in digestion for pets. It is typically administered as a tincture or in capsule form.

Remember to consult with a veterinarian before giving your pet any herbal remedies, as they can provide guidance on appropriate dosages and potential interactions with medications. Additionally, monitor your pet's response to any herbal remedy and report any adverse effects to your veterinarian.

Sustainable Herbal Practices

Sustainable herbal practices are a set of methods and principles designed to promote environmentally friendly and responsible use of medicinal and culinary herbs. These practices aim to maintain the natural balance of ecosystems, preserve plant biodiversity, and ensure the availability of herbs for future generations. Here's a more detailed explanation of some key principles of sustainable herbal practices.

1. Ethical Wildcrafting: When collecting herbs from their natural habitats, it is crucial to do so responsibly. This involves taking only what you need, leaving enough for the plant to regenerate, and ensuring that the species is not endangered. It's essential to respect local laws and regulations and avoid over-harvesting, which can lead to depletion of valuable plant resources.

2. Organic Cultivation: Growing herbs using organic methods helps to reduce the negative impacts of conventional agriculture on the environment. By avoiding synthetic pesticides and fertilisers, organic cultivation supports soil health, maintains biodiversity, and minimises harmful runoff into local waterways. Instead, natural compost and pest control methods are used to nourish and protect herb gardens.

3. Seed Saving and Plant Propagation: Preserving heirloom seeds and propagating plants is vital for maintaining genetic diversity among herbs. This practice also allows for the continuation of traditional herbal knowledge and contributes to a more resilient plant population in the face of environmental challenges.

4. **Water Conservation:** Implementing water-saving techniques such as drip irrigation or rainwater harvesting can significantly reduce the amount of water needed for herb gardens. Efficient water management is important in protecting this valuable natural resource and minimising the environmental impact of herb cultivation.

5. **Companion Planting:** Planting herbs alongside other plants can create a mutually beneficial environment by promoting natural pest control and improving the growth of neighbouring plants. This practice can help maintain a balanced ecosystem, reduce the need for synthetic pesticides, and contribute to overall plant health.

6. **Educating and Collaborating:** Sharing knowledge and collaborating with local communities, herbalists, and farmers is essential for promoting sustainable herbal practices. Building strong connections between people and plants encourages the responsible use and stewardship of these valuable resources.

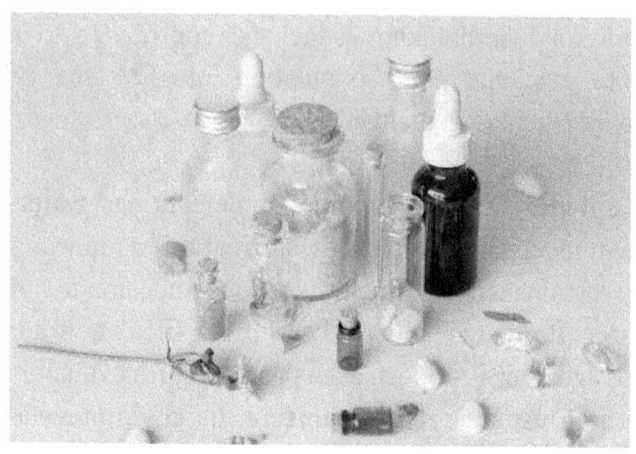

Adopting these sustainable herbal practices, individuals and communities can support the health of ecosystems and ensure the ongoing availability of medicinal and culinary herbs. This holistic approach to herbalism fosters a deeper connection with nature and contributes to a healthier, more resilient planet.

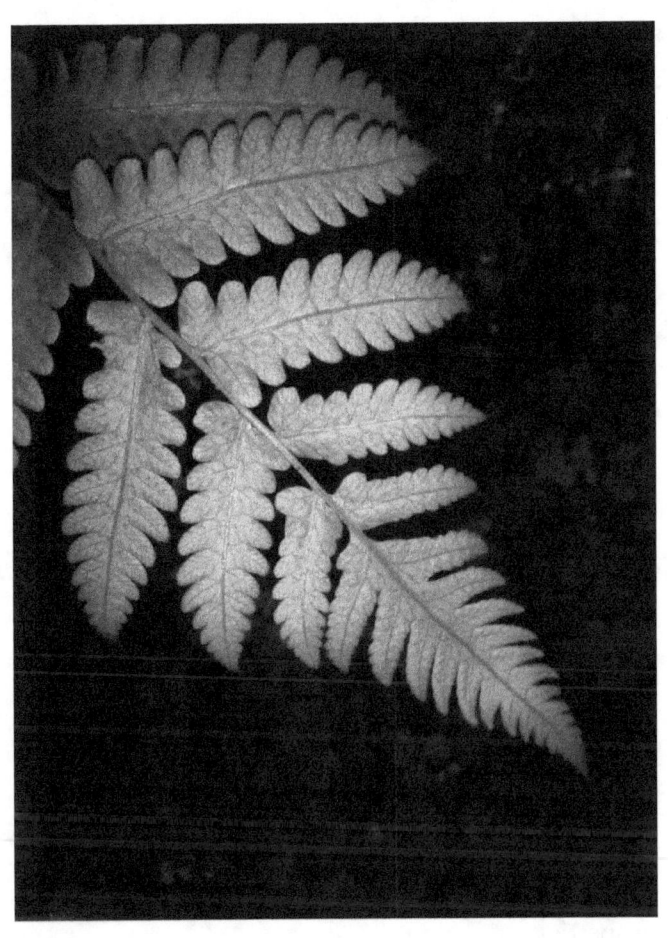

Chapter 15: Advanced Herbal Medicine

Clinical Applications of Herbal Medicine

Clinical applications of herbal medicine involve using plant-based remedies for the prevention and treatment of various health conditions. These applications have gained increasing recognition due to the growing interest in natural, alternative, and complementary therapies. Here's a closer look at some clinical areas where herbal medicine is commonly applied.

1. Pain Management: Herbal remedies such as turmeric, ginger, and willow bark have been used to alleviate pain and inflammation. These herbs contain compounds like curcumin, gingerol, and salicin, which possess analgesic and anti-inflammatory properties.

2. Digestive Health: Peppermint, chamomile, and ginger are examples of herbs commonly used to address digestive issues. They can help relieve symptoms of indigestion, bloating, and gas.

3. Mental Health: Herbs such as St. John's wort, valerian root, and lavender are known for their potential benefits in managing symptoms of anxiety, depression, and insomnia. They act on neurotransmitters and promote relaxation, helping to improve mood and sleep.

4. Cardiovascular Health: Herbs like garlic, hawthorn, and Terminalia arjuna have been studied for their potential in improving cardiovascular health. They possess cholesterol-lowering, antioxidant, and anti-inflammatory properties, which may help prevent heart disease.

5. Respiratory Health: Plants like eucalyptus, peppermint, and thyme have traditionally been used to relieve respiratory symptoms such as coughs and congestion. Their aromatic compounds help open airways and reduce inflammation.

6. Women's Health: Herbs such as black cohosh, red clover, and dong quai have been used for managing menopausal symptoms and menstrual disorders. They contain phytoestrogens that mimic the effects of oestrogen in the body.

7. Immune System Support: Echinacea, elderberry, and astragalus are among the many herbs known for their immune-boosting properties. They can help prevent and fight infections by stimulating immune cells and enhancing the production of antibodies.

In clinical settings, healthcare providers may recommend herbal medicine in conjunction with conventional treatments to enhance therapeutic outcomes. It's important to note that herbs can interact with medications and may not be suitable for everyone. It is important to consult with a qualified healthcare provider before incorporating herbal remedies into a treatment plan.

Herbal Formulations and Blends

Herbal formulations and blends involve combining two or more herbs to create a synergistic mixture that offers enhanced therapeutic benefits. This practice allows herbalists to address multiple aspects of a health condition and tailor remedies to individual needs. There are several types of herbal formulations and blends.

1. Simple Herbal Blends: These combine a small number of herbs with similar properties or actions to target a specific health concern. For example, a blend of chamomile, lavender, and passionflower could be used to promote relaxation and improve sleep.

2. Complex Herbal Formulas: These involve a larger number of herbs carefully selected to address multiple facets of a health issue. They may include herbs with complementary, opposing, or synergistic actions to enhance the overall efficacy and reduce potential side effects.

3. Traditional Formulas: These formulations are based on time-tested recipes passed down through generations or derived from ancient medicinal systems like Traditional Chinese Medicine or Ayurveda. Examples include the famous Chinese formula "Yin Qiao San" used to support immune health during the early stages of colds and flu.

4. Proprietary Blends: These are unique formulas created by individual herbalists or companies. They often contain a specific combination of herbs and may be trademarked or protected as intellectual property.

5. Customised Formulas: These are tailored to individual patients after thorough consultation with a trained herbalist or healthcare provider. They consider a person's unique symptoms, health history, and personal preferences to create a targeted, personalised remedy.

When preparing herbal formulations and blends, herbalists may use various extraction methods, such as teas, tinctures, capsules, or topical applications. Factors like herb potency, dosage, and potential interactions are carefully considered to ensure safety and efficacy.

Keep in mind that while herbal formulations and blends can offer many benefits, they should be used with caution and under the guidance of a qualified professional.

Research and Future of Herbal Medicine

Herbal medicine research has grown significantly in recent years, reflecting the increased interest in natural health solutions. This research encompasses various areas, including herbal pharmacology, drug discovery, and clinical applications. Here's a look at the current state and future directions of herbal medicine research.

1. Herbal Pharmacology: Researchers are actively studying the active compounds and mechanisms of action of various medicinal herbs. This helps to understand their effects on the human body and identify potential therapeutic applications.

2. Drug Discovery: Herbal medicine has become an essential source of novel drug discovery. Scientists are identifying and isolating bioactive compounds from plants, which can be developed into effective medications for various health conditions.

3. Clinical Trials: Randomized controlled trials are being conducted to evaluate the safety and efficacy of herbal remedies for specific health conditions. This evidence-based approach helps to determine which herbal therapies are effective and safe for broader clinical applications.

4. Quality Control and Standardization: Research focuses on developing better methods for ensuring the quality, consistency, and safety of herbal products. This includes establishing standardised extraction methods, determining optimal dosages, and identifying potential herb-drug interactions.

5. Personalised Medicine: Future research in herbal medicine may explore ways to tailor herbal therapies to individual patients, considering genetic variations, lifestyle factors, and unique health needs.

6. Sustainability and Conservation: Efforts are being made to ensure sustainable sourcing and cultivation practices for medicinal herbs. This helps to protect endangered species, preserve biodiversity, and secure the availability of herbs for future generations.

The future of herbal medicine holds great potential as research continues to deepen our understanding of the therapeutic benefits and applications of medicinal plants. This progress, combined with advancements in science and technology, will likely lead to improved herbal remedies and integrative healthcare approaches that enhance overall well-being.

Resources and Further Reading

here is a revised list of online resources and websites related to herbal medicine:

Websites and Online Publications:

1. American Botanical Council: https://abc.herbalgram.org/ A leading nonprofit organization providing research, education, and advocacy for herbal medicine.

2. Herbal Library: https://www.herbal-library.com/ A comprehensive digital library with extensive information on herbal medicine, including monographs, articles, and books.

3. Herbal Medicine:
https://www.mdpi.com/journal/herbs A peer-reviewed open-access journal dedicated to herbal medicine research and clinical applications.

4. National Center for Complementary and Integrative Health (NCCIH):
https://www.nccih.nih.gov/health/herbs-at-a-glance
A US government website providing evidence-based information on various herbs and their uses.

For more Resources and Further Reading consider the following

1. HerbMed:
https://herbmed.org/

A free online resource providing scientific and clinical information on herbal medicines, provided by the American Botanical Council and the National Center for Natural Products Research.

2. **The Herbal Resource:** https://www.herbal-supplement-resource.com/ A website with detailed articles on herbal supplements, their benefits, potential side effects, and interactions.

3. **Dr. Weil's Herbal Remedies:** https://www.drweil.com/health-wellness/herbs-supplements/ A collection of articles, videos, and resources on herbal remedies by renowned integrative medicine expert Dr. Andrew Weil.

Professional Organizations:

1. **American Herbalists Guild:** https://www.americanherbalistsguild.com/ A professional organization representing herbal practitioners, providing education and promoting herbal medicine.
2. **National Institute of Medical Herbalists:** https://www.nimh.org.uk/ A UK-based organization representing herbal medicine practitioners, offering resources and promoting professional standards.

Educational Programs:

1. **Herbal Academy:** https://theherbalacademy.com/ A comprehensive online educational platform offering various courses and programs in herbal medicine.

2. **Chestnut School of Herbal Medicine:** https://chestnutherbs.com/ An online herbal medicine school providing in-depth courses and programs for aspiring herbalists.

Always consult reputable sources and healthcare professionals when seeking information on herbal medicine.

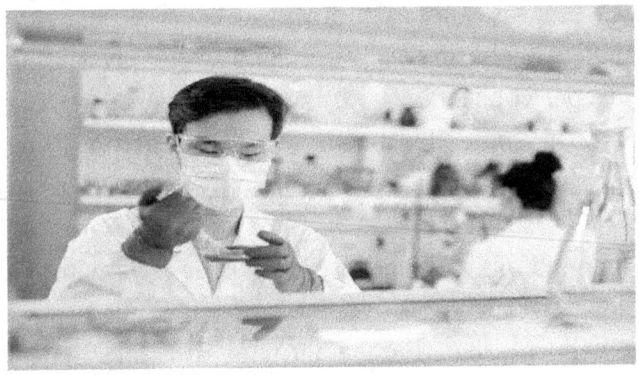

CONCLUSION

The journey through "The Book of Natural Medicine and Herbal Remedies: A Guide to Herbal Health and Cultivating Wellness" has unveiled the timeless wisdom and astounding potential of nature's gifts in promoting our health and well-being. embracing the holistic practices of herbalism, aromatherapy, yoga, meditation, and other natural therapies, we can tap into the Earth's abundant resources and enhance our lives in profound ways.

As we have explored an array of medicinal plants, essential oils, and herbal remedies, it is clear that these treasures hold the power to nourish, heal, and rejuvenate our bodies, minds, and spirits. Nurturing a deeper connection with the natural world, we can foster a more balanced, vibrant, and fulfilling existence for ourselves and our loved ones.

This guide has sought to empower readers with the knowledge and tools to embark on a lifelong journey of wellness, rooted in the harmony of nature. As we continue to learn and grow together, let us remember that the path to true health begins with the understanding that our well-being is intrinsically linked to the health of our planet. By honouring the Earth and its bountiful gifts, we can cultivate a thriving, sustainable future for generations to come.

May your journey through the realm of natural medicine and herbal remedies be filled with the joy of discovery, the wisdom of the ages, and the vibrant energy of life itself.

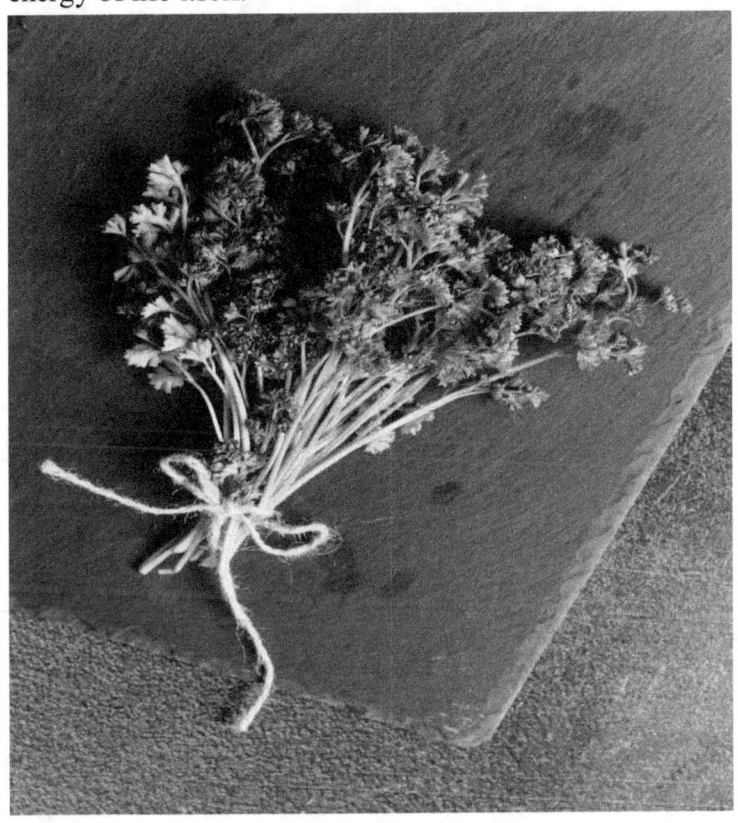

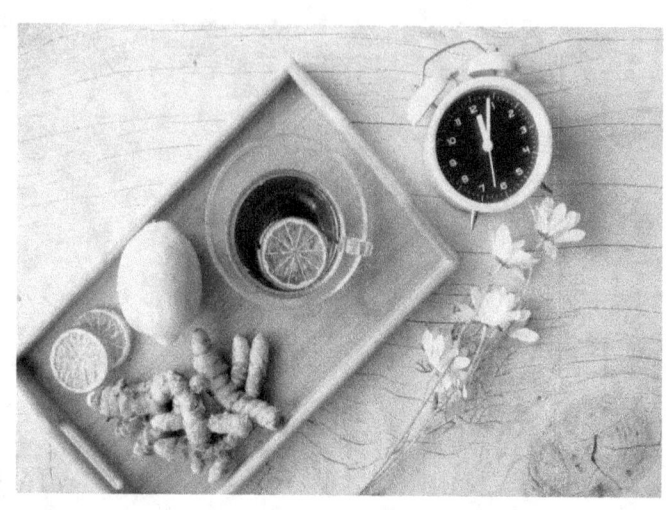